# Orthorexia Nervosa

'If any clinician, scientist or simply an interested person is looking for a comprehensive text regarding orthorexia nervosa, this recent book by Anna Brytek-Matera may be your answer. Professor Brytek-Matera offers a comprehensive review of this important topic with significant clinical insights. She follows the thread of this pattern of behaviour from normative efforts to attain healthy eating all the way to comparisons to anorexia nervosa and a variety of other psychiatric conditions. Of particular interest, she invited a handful of experts in behavioural health and eating disorders to offer commentary on the topic, which adds perspective. In general, I think this is an excellent contribution to the literature about eating disorders, and mental health, regarding this often misunderstood behavioural construct.'

**Stephen Wonderlich, Ph.D.**
Vice President, Chief of Behavioral Health Research – Sanford Fargo; Chester Fritz Distinguished Professor; University of North Dakota School of Medicine and Health Sciences

# Orthorexia Nervosa

## Current Understanding and Perspectives

**Anna Brytek-Matera**
University of Wrocław

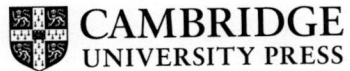

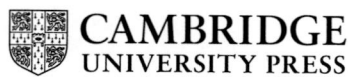

Shaftesbury Road, Cambridge CB2 8EA, United Kingdom

One Liberty Plaza, 20th Floor, New York, NY 10006, USA

477 Williamstown Road, Port Melbourne, VIC 3207, Australia

314–321, 3rd Floor, Plot 3, Splendor Forum, Jasola District Centre, New Delhi – 110025, India

103 Penang Road, #05–06/07, Visioncrest Commercial, Singapore 238467

Cambridge University Press is part of Cambridge University Press & Assessment, a department of the University of Cambridge.

We share the University's mission to contribute to society through the pursuit of education, learning and research at the highest international levels of excellence.

www.cambridge.org
Information on this title: www.cambridge.org/9781009216418

DOI: 10.1017/9781009216432

© Cambridge University Press & Assessment 2024

First published 2024

A catalogue record for this publication is available from the British Library.

Library of Congress Cataloging-in-Publication Data
Names: Brytek-Matera, Anna, author.
Title: Orthorexia nervosa : current understanding and perspectives / Anna Brytek-Matera.
Description: Cambridge, United Kingdom ; New York, NY : Cambridge University Press, 2024. | Includes bibliographical references and index.
Identifiers: LCCN 2024007995 (print) | LCCN 2024007996 (ebook) | ISBN 9781009216418 (paperback) | ISBN 9781009216432 (ebook)
Subjects: MESH: Orthorexia Nervosa | Diet, Healthy – adverse effects
Classification: LCC RA784 (print) | LCC RA784 (ebook) | NLM WM 175 | DDC 613.2–dc23/eng/20240524
LC record available at https://lccn.loc.gov/2024007995
LC ebook record available at https://lccn.loc.gov/2024007996

ISBN 978-1-009-21641-8 Paperback

To Mikołaj and Leon
with love

# Contents

# Foreword

In the early 2000s there was a 'mad cow' epidemic in Europe. Citizens, especially in Italy, were particularly affected and an attitude of fear developed when comparing certain foods, and beef in particular.

A collective orthorexic attitude manifested itself in the search for 'healthy' food that could not be a vehicle for substances or microorganisms dangerous to human health.

In our research unit we decided to study this phenomenon, which had already been described by Steve Bratman a few years earlier but had not received adequate attention or stimulated significant research.

We proposed a diagnostic tool (the ORTO-15) that was validated considering a definition of orthorexia nervosa based on the concept that this is a disorder characterised by a combination of eating behaviours (assessed using a questionnaire on eating habits, with special emphasis on the choices between food normally considered 'healthy' and 'unhealthy') and obsessive-phobic personality traits (evaluated administering the Minnesota Multiphasic Personality Inventory).

Despite the changes over time in the definition of the concept of orthorexia and some limitations from the point of view of the psychometric properties of this diagnostic tool, ORTO-15 kicked off important research in this field including the proposal of other diagnostic tools, the analysis of the clinical, psychological and functional characteristics of individuals who exhibited orthorexia, and finally the establishment of a consensus network to agree upon the definition and the diagnostic criteria for orthorexia nervosa.

Professor Brytek-Matera was immediately one of the principal researchers who contributed to the development of the concept of orthorexia by validating a version of the ORTO-15 for the Polish population. She addressed some specific aspects such as the relationship between disordered eating attitudes or vegetarian/vegan diet and orthorexia, and the interaction between orthorexia and the psychological phenotype (personality traits, self-esteem, obsessive-compulsive disorders, alexithymia and emotional dysregulation).

The book *Orthorexia Nervosa: Current Understanding and Perspectives* written by Professor Anna Brytek-Matera exhaustively explains the results of research in the field of orthorexia conducted by the scientific community and by Professor Brytek-Matera in particular. It represents an extremely interesting up-to-date document focusing on many aspects of research in this field.

It addresses general aspects (healthy and sustainable diets and behaviours, and dietary patterns) introducing the clinical description of orthorexia nervosa (diagnostic overview, comparison between orthorexia nervosa and eating disorders, obsessive-compulsive disorder or avoidant/restrictive food intake disorder). Another important topic developed in the book is the assessment and prevalence of orthorexia nervosa by evaluating the strengths and the limits of the diagnostic tools that have been proposed in the literature over the years. The multidimensional characteristics of orthorexia nervosa are also tackled, with particular attention to psychological (self-esteem, personality traits, body image and emotion regulation) and nutritional (dietary patterns and dieting trends) characteristics.

Finally, there is a comprehensive updated analysis of two decades of research on orthorexia nervosa focusing on the results in different populations (Western societies, clinical and non-clinical samples, and health professionals) and leading to a look at future directions for this newly proposed diagnosis belonging to eating disorders that may have severe mental and physical consequences.

Thus, it is a book that was missing and can definitely be a reference for those who deal with, from a clinical and research point of view, orthorexia nervosa.

Professor Lorenzo Maria Donini
*Sapienza University*

# Preface

Since the late 1990s, when Steven Bratman described 'the obsession with healthful eating' for the first time, scientific interest in orthorexia nervosa has grown from a handful of papers being published every year from 2004 to more than 70 in 2023 (PubMed search). For two decades, academics, researchers and clinicians across the globe have been wondering about the status of orthorexia nervosa. Is orthorexia nervosa a distinct clinical disorder, a variant of other conditions sharing traits with anorexia nervosa and/or obsessive-compulsive disorder? Should orthorexia nervosa likely be clinically categorised as an avoidant/restrictive food intake disorder? Or finally, perhaps it should be perceived as a healthy lifestyle?

Eating behaviour can appear on a continuum that ranges from a normative eating behaviour at one pole to a pathological one at the other. I do believe that orthorexia nervosa is a pathological condition since focusing on extreme healthy eating norms and behaviours (and thereby reduced food intake) to achieve optimal health negatively affects psychosocial functioning. I do not share the opinion that orthorexia nervosa is a social phenomenon or a healthy lifestyle. In my view, the point at which an eating behaviour becomes disordered is when, in addition to dietary restriction, obsessive thoughts together with negative feelings (e.g. induced distress or guilt) result in disturbing everyday functioning in the family, social and professional areas of an individual's life. Without a doubt, orthorexic behaviours, even if they eventuate from a healthy interest in nutrition, are not health-promoting. I do believe that individuals with extremely healthy eating patterns require support, help and treatment.

This book aims to systematise and present complex knowledge about orthorexia nervosa by characterising the various aspects of this unhealthy eating behaviour. Part I gives an overview of healthy dietary pattern recommendations to illustrate objective information on a healthy diet. Part II presents diagnostic criteria sets for orthorexia nervosa to depict key features of the condition, as well as the divergence and overlap of orthorexia nervosa and other mental disorders, namely anorexia nervosa, obsessive-compulsive disorder and avoidant/restrictive food intake disorder, to enable a differential diagnosis. Part III provides brief descriptions of the most frequently used self-reported questionnaires to outline those that seem suitable as self-assessment tools to measure orthorexia nervosa and are promising in research and clinical settings. Part IV emphasises the significance of psychological and nutritional characteristics of orthorexia nervosa to gain better insight into the construct of orthorexia nervosa. Part V focuses on research findings on orthorexia nervosa in both non-clinical and clinical samples to provide the current state of knowledge on orthorexia nervosa. Finally, Part VI outlines several future directions for orthorexia nervosa. This book also includes commentaries by invited international experts who provide valuable insights on orthorexia nervosa.

# Acknowledgements

*Science and everyday life cannot and should not be separated.*
*Science, for me, gives a partial explanation of life.*
*In so far as it goes, it is based on fact, experience, and experiment …*
*I agree that faith is essential to success in life ….*
*In my view, all that is necessary for faith is the belief that by doing our best,*
*we shall come nearer to success and that success in our aims*
*(the improvement of a lot of mankind, present and future) is worth attaining.*

Rosalind Franklin in a letter to Ellis Franklin (1940)

I want to extend a special note of appreciation to professors Marle Alvarenga, Phillipa Hay and Thom Dunn, and doctors Caterina Novara, Hana Zickgraf, Jinbo He and Adrian Meule for accepting my invitation and sharing their views and expertise.

I would not have been able to work on this book without the resources from my loving family. I want to thank my parents, who have encouraged me to pursue my aspirations and strive for my goals (in each step of my academic career). This book would not have been possible without the support of my husband, Marcin, whose understanding has been invaluable, especially throughout the process of writing this book. Special thanks go to my dear sons, Mikołaj and Leon, who taught me to appreciate the little moments and made me realise that even though being a mother is sometimes difficult, it is the most crucial role in my life.

# About the Author

Anna Brytek-Matera, PhD is Professor of Medical and Health Sciences at the Institute of Psychology at the University of Wrocław, Poland, where she serves as Head of the Nutritional Psychology Unit, Eating Behavior Laboratory (EAT Lab) and Postgraduate Studies in Psychodietetics. She completed a Master of Cultural Studies and a Master of Psychology at the University of Silesia, Poland. She has been selected as the French Government Scholarship laureate (Cotutelle) and was awarded a doctoral degree in Psychology at Paul Verlaine University – Metz, France. Professor Anna Brytek-Matera is the author and co-author of more than 150 scientific publications on orthorexia nervosa, eating disorders and eating behaviour, including eight books (e.g. *Eating Disorders*, 2021; *Psychodietetics*, 2020). She has been named in the top 2% of the world's most influential scientists (World's top 2% scientists 2021 and 2022 – The Single Year Impact). She serves on the editorial board for *Eating and Weight Disorders* and *Nutrients*. Throughout her career, she has been involved with research around orthorexia nervosa, eating disorders and weight-related behaviour. Her research has been supported by grants from the Polish National Agency for Academic Exchange, National Science Center, Ministry of Science and Higher Education, Foundation for Polish Science, and Fondation Maison des Sciences de l'Homme, France. She has given guest lectures at universities around the United States of America (Stanford University), Asia (The University of Tokyo), Australia (Western Sydney University) and Europe (University of Nantes, University of Bordeaux, University of Padova, University of Pavia, University of West London).

Professor Anna Brytek-Matera represents the scientist-practitioner model. Besides her scientific research activity, as a cognitive behavioural therapist she works with patients with eating disorders.

# Part I
# Dieting Trends and Health

# 1 Healthy and Sustainable Diet

## 1.1 Healthy Diet

Diet is one of the 'big three' modifiable health behaviours (together with sleep and physical activity) (Wickham et al., 2020). The World Health Organization (WHO, 2020) defines a healthy diet as achieving energy balance, limiting energy intake from total fats, free sugars and salt and increasing consumption of fruits and vegetables, legumes, whole grains and nuts. Regular consumption of a wide variety of foods from key food groups in the right proportions and consuming the right amount of food and drink are conducive to achieving, improving, enhancing and maintaining a healthy body weight (National Health Service (NHS), 2022) and health by reduction of the risk of chronic illness (WHO, 2020). A healthy diet should ensure an adequate intake of macronutrients (i.e. carbohydrates, proteins and lipids) that provide a significant contribution to the caloric intake and micronutrients (i.e. vitamins and minerals) that are considered crucial for the health and vital functions of the human body. In addition, it should provide a diversity of foods of high nutritional quality, be safe to consume (High Level Panel of Experts (HLPE), 2017) and reduce the risk for non-communicable diseases (WHO, 2018, 2020) (see Table 1.1). A balanced, adequate and varied diet is essential for health and well-being (WHO, 2020).

The content of a diversified, balanced and healthy diet varies depending on individual needs and characteristics (e.g. age, sex, lifestyle and degree of physical activity), locally available foods, dietary customs, cultural context and other considerations (e.g. geographical and environmental aspects). However, the basic principles of a healthy diet remain the same for everyone (WHO, 2020). The World Health Organization's recommendations for maintaining a healthy diet (WHO, 2018, 2020), based on WHO Nutrition Guidance Expert Advisory Group work to date and prior expert consultations or reports on diet and disease, are presented in Table 1.2.

The Eatwell Guide, produced by the United Kingdom's National Health Service (Public Health England, 2016a, 2016b), represents food-based dietary guidelines by giving a visual representation of the different types and the appropriate proportions of foods and drinks required to achieve a balanced diet and improve dietary health. The guidelines are directed at the general population from the age of two years. The Eatwell Guide is based on five food groups, namely fruit and vegetables (weight of food: 40%), potatoes, bread, rice, pasta and other starchy carbohydrates

Table 1.1 Key elements of a healthy diet and their characteristics

| Key element | Characteristics |
| --- | --- |
| Quantity | • Adequate food energy to maintain life, support physical activity and achieve and maintain a healthy body weight.<br>• Adequate amounts of macro- and micronutrients to meet individual nutrition and health needs.<br>• Limitation of overconsumption, particularly energy-dense, nutrient-poor food (high in saturated and trans-fats, added sugars and salt). |
| Diversity | • Variety of nutrient-dense foods from basic food groupings, including vegetables, fruits, whole grains and cereals, dairy foods and animal- and plant-based protein foods. |
| Quality | • Needed amounts of macro- and micronutrients.<br>• Foods should not contain unspecified or unhealthy additives such as trans-fats. |
| Safety | • Foods and beverages being safe to consume. |

Source: Based on High Level Panel of Experts (HLPE, 2017).

Table 1.2 The World Health Organization's current recommendations for a healthy diet in adults

| Recommendations | Objective |
| --- | --- |
| • Eating a variety of whole (i.e. unprocessed) and fresh foods, including staple foods (e.g. cereals such as wheat, barley, rye, maize and rice; or starchy tubers or roots such as potato, yam, taro and cassava), legumes (e.g. lentils and beans), vegetables, fruit and foods from animal sources (e.g. meat, fish, eggs and milk).<br>• Obtaining the largest amount of energy from carbohydrates, mainly through legumes and wholegrain cereals. | Obtaining the right amounts of essential nutrients, that is, protein, vitamins and minerals, and balancing energy intake with expenditure. |
| • Consuming at least 400 g of vegetables and fruit per day. | Reducing the risk of non-communicable diseases and helping to ensure an adequate daily intake of vitamins, minerals, dietary fibre, plant protein and antioxidants. |

Table 1.2 (cont.)

| Recommendations | Objective |
| --- | --- |
| • Limiting total fat intake to not exceeding 30% of total energy intake. | Preventing unhealthy weight gain. |
| • Limiting intake of saturated fats to less than 10% of total energy intake. | |
| • Limiting trans-fat intake to less than 1% of total energy intake, shifting fat consumption away from saturated fats and trans-fats to unsaturated fats and towards eliminating industrially produced trans-fats. | |
| • Limiting intake of free sugars to less than 10% of total energy intake. A further reduction to less than 5% of total energy intake is suggested for additional health benefits. | Preventing high blood pressure and protecting against heart disease and stroke. |
| • Keeping salt intake to less than 5 g per day (equivalent to sodium intake of less than 2 g per day). | |

Source: Based on World Health Organization (WHO, 2018, 2020).

(38%), beans, pulses, fish, eggs, meat and other proteins (12%), dairy and alternatives (8%) and oils and spreads (1%), and illustrates the proportion that each food group should contribute to a healthy balanced diet (Public Health England, 2016a) (see Figure 1.1). The proportions shown are representative of food consumption over a day or even a week, not necessarily at each mealtime.

Individuals decide on multiple food choices each day. Many factors, including genes, influence these choices, as do learned experiences with food and the broader physical, social and cultural environment (Monterrosa et al., 2020). Awareness of the importance of balanced nutrition is an essential factor that may influence dietary choices (Alkerwi et al., 2015). Both individual determinants of personal food choices, including one's physiological state (e.g. innate preferences for sweet and aversion for bitter tastes), food preference, nutritional knowledge, perception of healthy eating (public understanding of and opinion – views, attitudes and beliefs – about healthy eating), psychological factors (e.g. emotions, mood, well-being), and collective determinants of eating behaviour, including interpersonal environment (e.g. family, peers), physical environment, economic environment, social environment and healthy public policy, determine healthy eating (Raine, 2005) (see Figure 1.2).

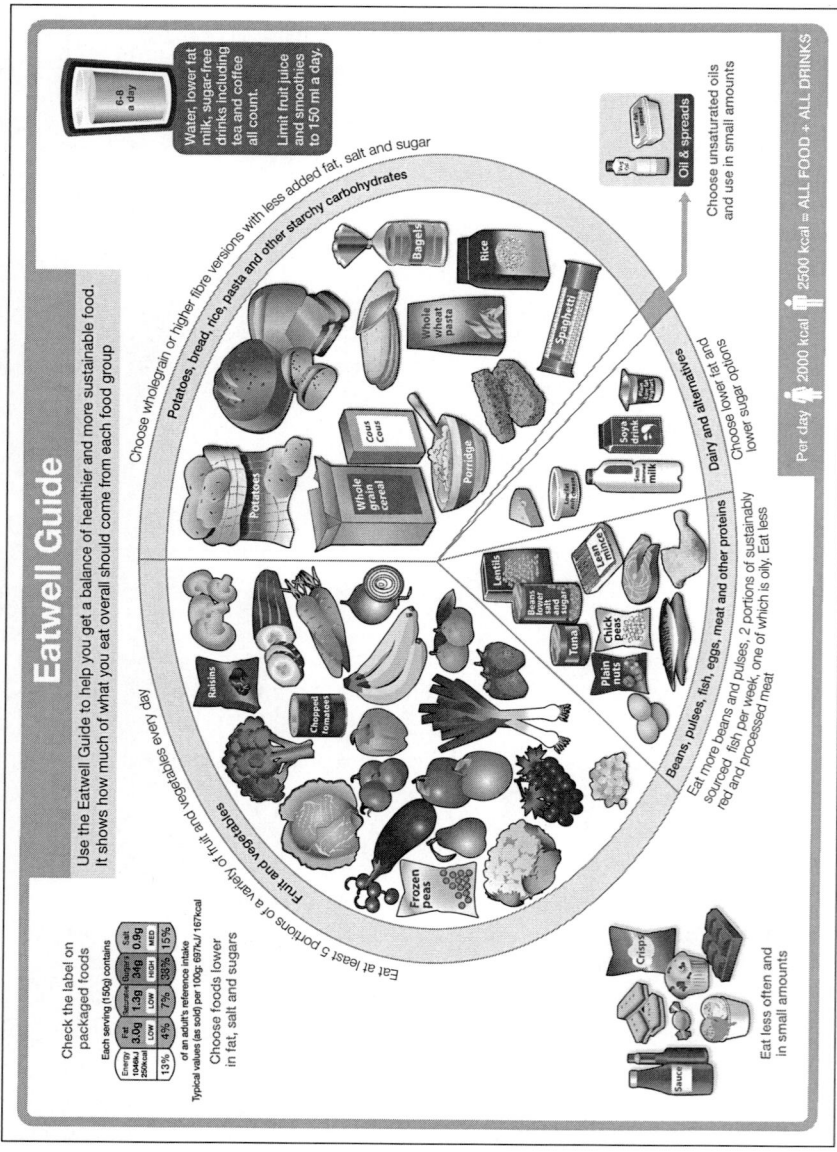

**Figure 1.1** Food groups in a healthy and balanced diet: Eatwell Guide.
Source: UK Health Security Agency in association with the Welsh Government, Food Standards Scotland and the Food Standards Agency in Northern Ireland. Reproduced with permission.

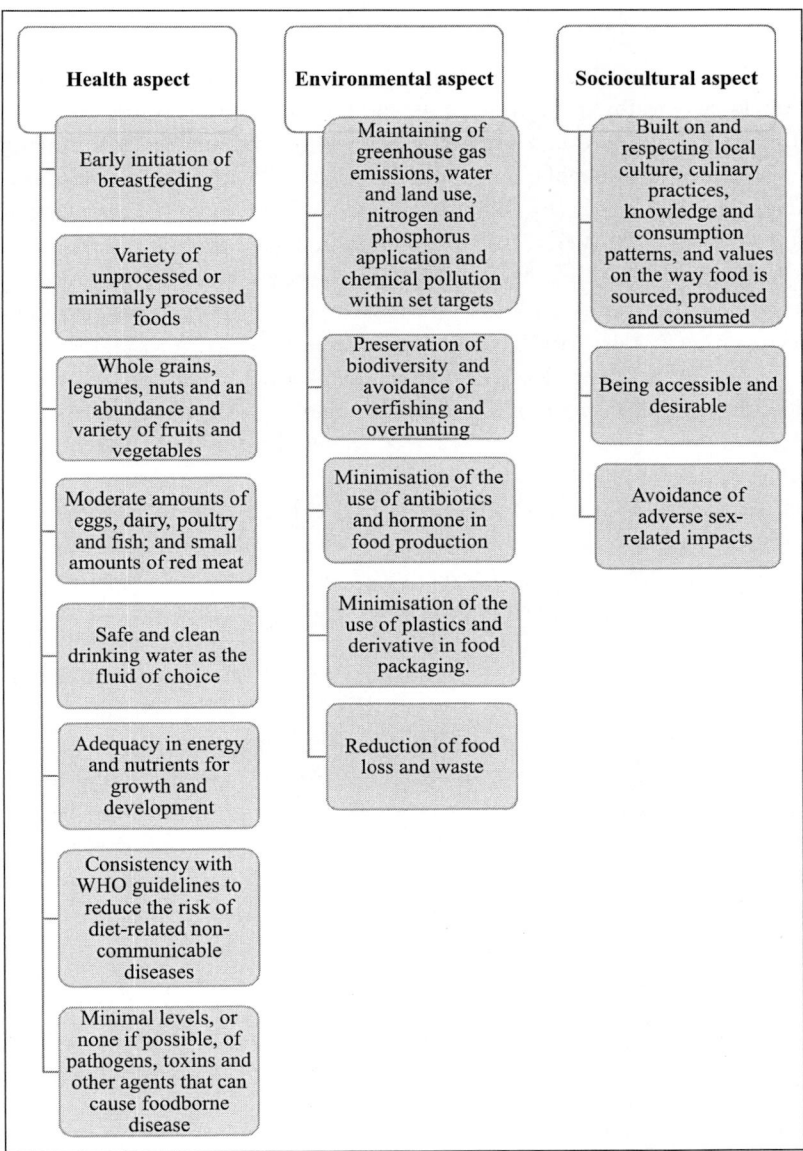

**Figure 1.2** Guiding principles for sustainable healthy diets according to the Food and Agriculture Organization (FAO) and WHO.
Source: Based on Food and Agriculture Organization and World Health Organization (2019).

## 1.2 Sustainable Healthy Diets

Sustainable healthy diets are dietary patterns that promote all dimensions of individuals' health and (physical, mental and social) well-being, have low environmental pressure and impact, are accessible, affordable, nutritionally adequate, safe and equitable, as well as being culturally acceptable, while optimising natural and human resources (Food and Agriculture Organization (FAO), 2012; FAO & WHO, 2019). The definition produced by the FAO and the WHO placed health at the forefront of consideration while still underscoring the need to consider other aspects, whereas in the previous definition (Burlingame & Dernini, 2012), economic and environmental goals of diets were often given pre-eminence (Harrison et al., 2022). Health, environmental and socio-cultural aspects are dimensions of sustainable healthy diets that must be considered together to achieve sustainable healthy diets (FAO & WHO, 2019) (see Figure 1.3).

As the FAO and the WHO (FAO & WHO, 2019) clearly state, one of the actions required to make sustainable healthy diets available, accessible, affordable, safe and desirable is the development of national food-based dietary guidelines (that represent healthy diets in a culturally appropriate dietary pattern for the country in which they are designed) according to the principles presented in Figure 1.3 (FAO & WHO, 2019). It is also important to note that just because a diet is sustainable, it is not necessarily healthy (Hemler & Hu, 2019). Vegan and vegetarian diets typically have less environmental impact than diets containing meat (Melina et al., 2016), but a vegan eating many refined carbohydrates and added sugars could be at a greater risk for weight gain and chronic diseases than an omnivore consuming meat and a variety of healthy plant-based foods. Although it is possible to achieve a healthy and sustainable diet without becoming vegan or vegetarian, these dietary patterns, if comprised of high-quality plant foods and are appropriately planned to avoid deficiencies, can be nutritionally adequate for all stages of the life cycle (including infancy, pregnancy and older adulthood) and can reduce chronic disease risk (Melina et al., 2016).

## 1.3 Dietary Patterns

Diet evolves over time, being influenced by a variety of factors, including food-internal (e.g. sensory and perceptual features), individual (psychological, physical, neurological, cognitive; e.g. individual preferences and beliefs, knowledge and skills), social (e.g. income), economic (e.g. food prices) and environmental factors (e.g. time) that interact in a complex manner to shape

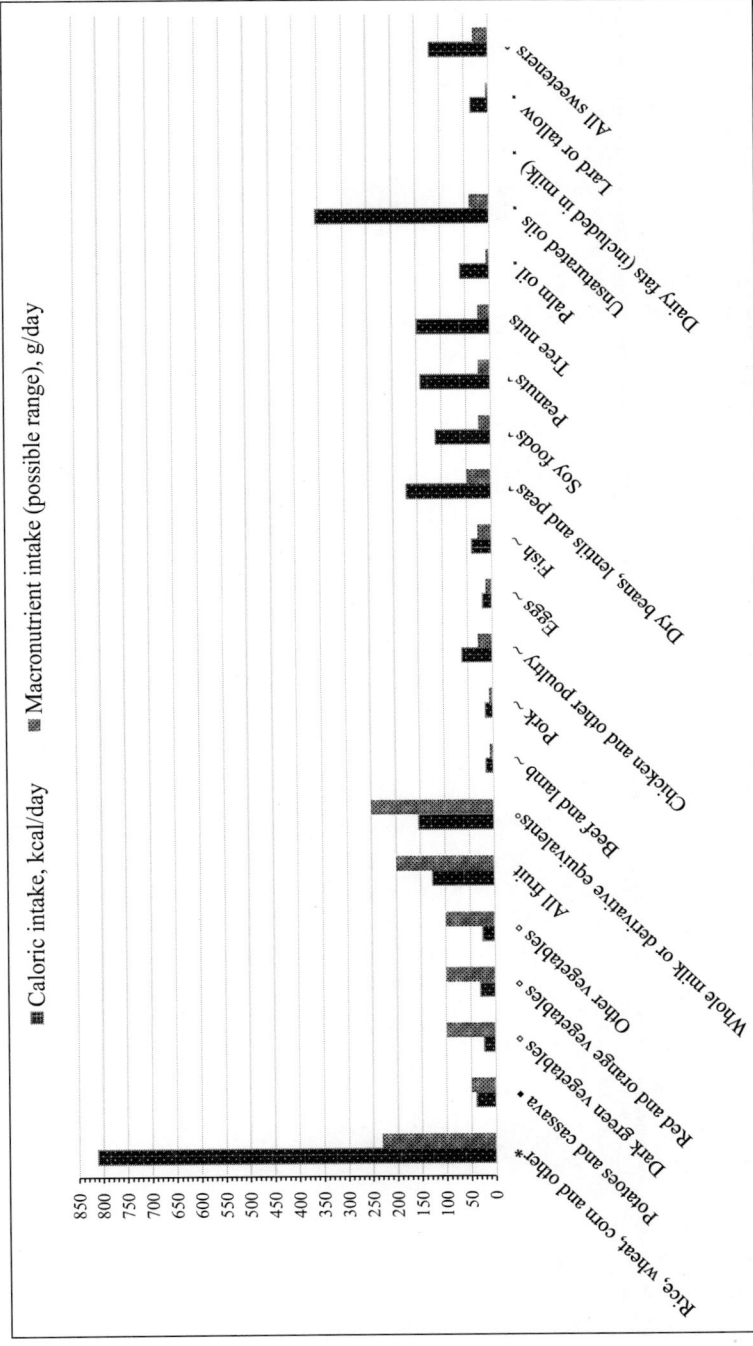

**Figure 1.3** Healthy reference diet for an intake of 2,500 kcal/day.

* Whole grains; • Tubers or starchy vegetables; □ Vegetables; ○ Daily foods; ~ Protein sources; ˄ Legumes; · Added fats; ˙ Added sugars

Source: Based on Willett et al. (2019).

individual dietary patterns (Chen & Antonelli, 2020). Dietary patterns can be defined as the quantities, proportions, variety or combination of different foods, drinks and nutrients in diets in relation to the five food groups of the Eatwell Guide, United Kingdom and the MyPlate, United States of America (fruit and vegetables, carbohydrates/grains, protein, fats and sugar, dairy products) (Timlin et al., 2020), and the frequency with which they are habitually consumed (Bouchey et al., 2020).

The number of diets available in the market is excessive. Therefore, it is worth knowing how to make an informed food choice. A recent report, 'Best Diets of 2023' by US News and World Report (2023), released 24 diets ranked by medical experts, nutritionists, dietitians, physicians and epidemiologists. The Mediterranean diet (number 1 for the sixth year in a row), the Dietary Approaches to Stop Hypertension (DASH) diet and the flexitarian diet remain the 'Best Overall Diets' and the 'Best Diets for Healthy Eating' of 2023 (4.6 out of 5 points, 4.5 out of 5 points and 4.3 out of 5 points, respectively). The Mediterranean diet is a territorial plant-based diet with little to moderate amounts of animal-sourced foods. It is characterised by an abundance of vegetables, fruits, nuts, legumes, seeds and fish, with liberal use of olive oil, a moderate amount of dairy foods and a low amount of red meat (Hachem et al., 2016). Strong scientific evidence showing the association of the Mediterranean diet with a significant reduction in total mortality, mortality from cardiovascular disease and cancer, and a lowered cancer risk has led to this dietary pattern being promoted in regions and dietary guidelines of countries far from its geographic origins (Hachem et al., 2016). It is worth noting that 10 years ago the Mediterranean diet was included on the Intangible Cultural Heritage List of the United Nations Educational, Scientific and Cultural Organization (UNESCO) by the Intergovernmental Committee of the Convention concerning the Intangible Heritage of Humanity (United Nations Educational Social and Cultural Organization, 2013, as cited in Subhan & Chan, 2016). Similar to the Mediterranean diet, the DASH diet incorporates fruits, vegetables, whole grains, fat-free/low-fat dairy, nuts and legumes, lean meat choices, limiting total and saturated fat, cholesterol, red and processed meats, sugar-sweetened beverages, sweets and added sugars and consuming reduced amounts of sodium (Chiavaroli et al., 2019). A flexitarian diet (also known as a semi-vegetarian diet) primarily (but not strictly) includes a vegetarian diet with the occasional inclusion of meat or fish (Derbyshire, 2017).

The EAT–Lancet reference diet (Willett et al., 2019) is the first global benchmark diet capable of sustaining health and protecting the planet at the same time, minimising chronic disease risks and maximising human well-being. It is rich in fruits and vegetables, with protein and fats sourced mainly from plant-based foods, unsaturated fish oils and carbohydrates from whole grains (see Figure 1.3). The healthy dietary pattern consists of ranges of intakes for each food group. For an individual, an optimal energy intake to maintain a healthy weight depends on body size and level of physical activity. The global average per capita energy intake has been estimated as 2,370 kcal per day (Hiç et al., 2016), ranging from 2,000 to 2,200 kcal per day for women to 2,800 kcal per day for men (Freedman et al., 2014). Therefore, 2,500 kcal per day has been used as a basis for different isocaloric dietary scenarios (i.e. having similar caloric values) (see Figure 1.4).

The idea of classifying foods as 'healthy' and 'unhealthy'[1] based on their nutrient composition (Lobstein & Davies, 2008) is still discussed, with a general lack of consensus. Some argue that no foods are inherently 'healthy' or 'unhealthy' and that all foods can be part of a healthy diet if consumed in moderation. More and more, there is a push to move from nutrient-specific or food-specific approaches to more holistic ones examining overall dietary

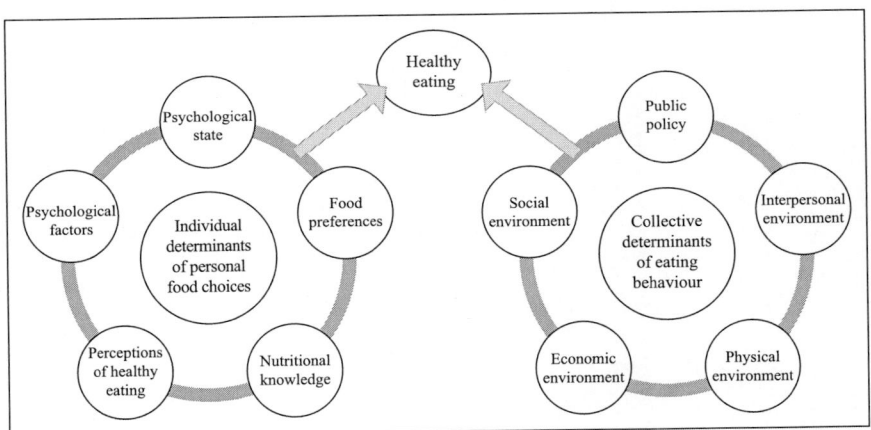

Figure 1.4 Determinants of healthy eating.
Source: Based on Raine (2005).

[1] Typically, an unhealthy diet is described as low in fruits, vegetables, whole grains, nuts and seeds, milk, fibre, calcium, seafood and fish high in omega-3 fatty acids, and polyunsaturated fatty acids, and diets high in red meat, processed meat (smoked, cured, salted or chemically preserved), sugar-sweetened beverages, trans-fats and sodium (GBD 2013 Risk Factors Collaborators et al., 2015). An unhealthy diet is considered as one of the leading risks for the global burden of disease, mainly for non-communicable diseases, such as cardiovascular diseases, diabetes and cancer (WHO, 2020), deaths and disability-adjusted life years lost (GBD 2013 Risk Factors Collaborators et al., 2015).

patterns (Mozaffarian & Ludwig, 2010). According to the Academy of Nutrition and Dietetics (Freeland-Graves et al., 2013), the total diet or overall pattern of food eaten is more important to a healthy diet than focusing on single foods or individual nutrients and labelling specific foods as 'good food' or 'bad food' that may foster unhealthy eating behaviours. Messages emphasising the total diet approach promote positive lifestyle changes (Freeland-Graves et al., 2013). In addition, focus on variety, moderation and proportionality in a healthy lifestyle are the key concepts for balancing food and beverage intake (Freeland-Graves et al., 2013). When making dietary recommendations, it is essential to emphasise overall dietary patterns rather than specific foods and nutrients to account for the synergistic effects of the total diet on health (Dietary Guidelines Advisory Committee, 2015).

# 2 Health Behaviours and Healthy Eating Interventions

## 2.1 Health Behaviours

Over the past decades, there has been an upsurge of interest in health and health behaviours. More precisely, this interest and efforts to change health behaviours emerged from the mid twentieth century onwards (Armstrong, 2009). Health behaviours (or health-related behaviour) have been defined as 'personal attributes such as beliefs, expectations, motives, values, perceptions, and other cognitive elements; personality characteristics including affective and emotional states and traits and overt behaviour patterns, actions, and habits that relate to health maintenance, to health restoration, and health improvement' (Gochman, 1997, p. 3). This means that not only observable, overt actions but also mental events and emotional states can be reported and measured. Health behaviours include a set of actions related to nutrition, addictive substances, movement and physical exercises (Havigerová, Dosedlová & Burešová, 2018). These behaviours may be intentional or unintentional, affect health directly or indirectly, and can promote or detract from the individual's health and physical and psychological well-being (Short & Mollborn, 2015) (Table 2.1).

Health-enhancing behaviour ('healthy' or 'healthful') and health-impairing behaviour ('unhealthy', 'risky' or 'health-compromising') can be thought of as dichotomies (positive versus negative). Health behaviours are increasingly considered multidimensional and embedded in health lifestyles, varying throughout life (Short & Mollborn, 2015). They are frequently discussed as individual-level behaviours but can also be measured for groups or populations. Health psychologist researchers attempt to explain between-individual variation (why do some people differ one from another in their behaviour; e.g. why are some people more likely to eat fruits and vegetables while others do not?) and within-individual variation (why does an individual's behaviour vary over time or across different settings; e.g. why does someone eat more sweets on some days or in some situations rather than in others?) in particular health behaviours using theories of health behaviour (Sutton, 2008).

Table 2.1 Examples of health behaviours promoting or detracting from the health

| Health-enhancing behaviour | Health-impairing behaviour |
| --- | --- |
| • Healthy diet (e.g. eating at least five portions of fruit and vegetables a day) | • Inappropriate eating habits (e.g. eating a diet high in saturated fat) |
| • Regular physical activity | • Sedentary living and lack of exercise |
| • Appropriate sleep regime | • Insufficient sleep |
| • Healthcare-seeking behaviours | • Excessive alcohol intake |
| • Participation in health screening examinations | • Risky sexual behaviour |
| • Adherence to prescribed medical treatments | • Substance use |
| | • Smoking |

## 2.2 Theories of Health Behaviour and Their Use in Healthy Eating Interventions

Interventions to change health-related behaviours may be more effective if grounded in appropriate theory (Davis et al., 2015). Several general models of the psychological determinants of health behaviours have been developed over the years (Table 2.2).

Models of individual health behaviour, such as the Health Belief Model, Theory of Reasoned Action/Theory of Planned Behaviour and models of interpersonal behaviour, such as Social Cognitive Theory, integrate the key influences on healthy behaviours (Conner & Norman, 2005). Importantly, these models focus on various health cognitions as key proximal determinants of health behaviours common across different health behaviours (Conner, 2019).

Health behavioural theories help understand dietary behaviours and develop intervention strategies. The recent review (Luo & Allman-Farinelli, 2021) on behavioural theory-based interventions for healthy eating has demonstrated that the Social Cognitive Theory was the most used and dominant over the past 20 years. Other behaviour change theories used in healthy eating interventions over the past two decades were the Theory of Planned Behaviour, the Health Belief Model, the Transtheoretical Model and the Self-determination Theory (Luo & Allman-Farinelli, 2021). Moreover, in the previous scoping review (Davis et al., 2015), the Social Cognitive Theory, the Transtheoretical Model of Change, the Theory of Planned Behaviour and the Information-Motivation-Behavioural-Skills Model have been identified as the most utilised theories that identified

Table 2.2 Classification of theories of health behaviour

| Classification | Characteristics | Example |
|---|---|---|
| By range of application | | |
| General theory | Applied to a wide range of behaviours, not simply health-related ones | Theory of Planned Behaviour |
| Health specific theory | Specific to health-related behaviours | Health Belief Model |
| Domain- or behaviour-specific theory | Narrow range of application | Health-promoting nutrition behaviours |
| By formal structure | | |
| Stage theory (stage-based theory) | Behaviour change involves movement through a sequence of discrete stages | Transtheoretical Model |
| Non-stage theory (continuum-based theory) | Behaviour change is a continuous process | Theory of Planned Behaviour |

Source: Based on Sutton (2008).

theories of behaviour and behaviour change of potential relevance to public health interventions in the discipline of psychology, sociology, anthropology and economics. In a systematic review of 19 randomised controlled trials of theory-informed dietetic interventions in primary healthcare settings (Rigby et al., 2020), the Social Cognitive Theory was found to be most commonly applied in interventions and to have significant intervention effects. Goal setting, problem-solving, social support and self-monitoring were the most commonly reported techniques (Rigby et al., 2020). The primary dietary behaviours targeted by the theory-based nutrition interventions included healthy eating patterns, an increase in fruit and/or vegetable intake, an increase in dairy, calcium and/or vitamin D food source intake, a decrease in dietary fat, a reduction of discretionary food intake and a decrease in sugar-sweetened beverage intake and others (e.g. decreasing snacking, increasing breakfasting, following a Mediterranean diet) (Luo & Allman-Farinelli, 2021). However, the previous meta-analysis (Prestwich et al., 2014) revealed that theory use (particularly the Social Cognitive Theory and the Transtheoretical Model) is unlikely to increase the effectiveness of intervention targeting physical activity and healthy eating. In addition, the authors (Prestwich et al., 2014) found that about 90% of interventions report that they are based on a behaviour change theory. However, most still fail to clearly describe their strategies to change an individual's dietary intake according to the theory.

# Highlights

• The definition and concept of healthy eating varies and changes, shaped by socio-cultural context (McDonald & Braun, 2022). In recent years, efforts have been made to define healthy and sustainable diets. A healthy diet should optimise health, defined broadly by the World Health Organization as complete physical, mental and social well-being, not just the absence of disease (Willett et al., 2019). A healthy diet emphasises the importance of having an appropriate calorie intake which consists of a variety of nutrient-dense foods and beverages including increasing intake of plant-based foods, consuming unsaturated rather than saturated or trans-fats and limiting the intake of animal source foods, refined grains, highly processed foods, added sugars, salt and foods of minimal nutritional value (Global Nutrition Report, 2020). The benefits of a healthy diet are reflected in lifelong health (WHO, 2020). The previous systematic review and dose-response meta-analysis of prospective studies (Molendijk et al., 2018) demonstrated that regular adherence to a high-quality diet (i.e. healthy/prudent or Mediterranean diet) is linked to a lower risk of depressive symptoms and improved mood. In addition, combining a healthy diet and regular physical activity behaviours and patterns is central to promoting overall health and preventing many chronic diseases (Dietary Guidelines Advisory Committee, 2015).

• To increase the effectiveness of nutrition education in promoting sensible food choices, appropriate behavioural theory and evidence-based strategies must be utilised. The social cognitive theories, particularly the Social Cognitive Theory, the Theory of Planned Behaviour and the Theory of Reasoned Action, are frequently and commonly cited in the eating domain (Tucunduva, Guerra & Barco Leme, 2016). They help explain, predict and understand dietary behaviours and design dietary interventions to promote dietary change (Conner & Norman, 2005). Empirical evidence suggests inconsistent findings for the effectiveness of theory-based dietary interventions. Dietary interventions underpinned by behaviour change theories and utilising various behaviour change techniques may be more effective at improving patient health outcomes than those without theoretical underpinnings (Rigby et al., 2020). In addition, rigorous interventions using behaviour change theory lead to better trial outcomes (improvement of fruit and vegetable consumption) (Timlin et al., 2020). On the other hand, the previous meta-analysis (Prestwich et al., 2014) provided evidence that interventions based on Social Cognitive Theory or the Transtheoretical Model were similarly effective and no more effective than interventions without a behaviour change theoretical framework. The effectiveness of interventions that use social cognitive theories to promote whole dietary patterns has been limited (Timlin et al., 2020).

• Healthy eating is essential and helpful to achieve and maintain good health (McDonald & Braun, 2022), but how people understand what healthy eating involves is more complex. The belief about healthy foods can vary from person to person. In some cases, what individuals broadly classify as 'healthy diets' may differ from the recommended dietary allowance offered by scientific nutrition or public health guidelines. This may blur the boundary between healthy and unhealthy practices (Lewthwaite & LaMarre, 2022), and uncertainties about the quality of the products create a 'specific' approach to food consumption. Many people strive to eat a healthier diet, believing that their conscious nutritional choice helps them (not hinders them) in achieving their dietary goals. Unfortunately, they often are unaware that their dietary restrictions intended to promote health can paradoxically lead to unhealthy consequences. When cognitions and worries about healthy nutrition lead to an accurate food selection or a correct diet that becomes an essential part of an individual's life, this attitude can become pathological and alter eating behaviour to important dietary restrictions and stereotyped eating (i.e. eating only certain foods and avoiding many others sometimes with a shortage of essential nutrients) and may cause impairment in important areas of functioning (e.g. social) or for health (Segura-Garcia et al., 2015). Thus, in some individuals, healthy eating may become unhealthy. Their preoccupation with healthy eating and interest in healthy attitudes and behaviours towards food may contribute to orthorexia nervosa manifested by the avoidance of all foods considered by the individuals to be unhealthy.

# Part II

# Clinical Description of Orthorexia Nervosa

# 3 Definition of Orthorexia Nervosa

## 3.1 Variety of Definitions

The term 'orthorexia nervosa' was coined by physician Dr Steven Bratman in the late 1990s in the United States. In the book '*Health food junkies. Orthorexia nervosa: overcoming the obsession with healthful eating*', the author proposed that 'orthorexia nervosa refers to a fixation on eating healthy food' (Bratman & Knight, 2000, p. 9). Despite 20 years of research and debate, as well as a variety of definitions, there is still no standard definition for orthorexia nervosa. The existence of an official definition of orthorexia nervosa remains crucial for several reasons: to know if its diagnosis should or should not be included in the classification systems, to distinguish between pathological and normal conditions and to recognise the condition that, as a result of its negative consequences, requires (medical or psychological) treatment (Telles-Correia, Saraiva & Gonçalves, 2018).

Orthorexia nervosa has been defined as a (persistent or exaggerated or obsessive or pathological or monoideistic) fixation, (pathological or extreme or unhealthy or maniacal) obsession, (extreme) concern, (extreme or overwhelming or excessive or time-consuming) preoccupation or extreme phobia of healthy food/healthy eating (Cena et al., 2019). In general terms, orthorexia nervosa could be described as 'an overvaluation and preoccupation with food quality and its impact on health' (Donini et al., 2022, p. 3696). Additionally, the lack of a commonly established definition of orthorexia nervosa makes the question of whether orthorexia nervosa could be a phenomenon by proxy (Cuzzolaro & Donini, 2016) difficult to answer.

### 3.1.1 Is the Etymology of the Term 'Orthorexia Nervosa' Accurate? 'Salussitomania': A New Proposition for Describing Preoccupation with Health and Healthy Eating

The name 'orthorexia nervosa' is derived from the Greek term ὀρθο- (ortho-), meaning 'right', 'true', 'correct' and ὄρεξις (orexis), meaning 'desire', 'longing', 'appetite' (Liddell & Scott, 1996). That means 'right appetite' whereas the Latin term 'nervosa' means 'nervous' or 'mental'. In 2002, Hans Nyman, in the article 'En rak fråga: Ortorexi rätt ord på fel sak?' [A direct question: Is orthorexia a correct word for a wrong concept?] emphasised that, etymologically, the term 'orthorexia' is hardly perfect. He accentuated that it is not primarily about the appetite but rather a 'mania' for a certain type of food. He proposed to consider three terms: 'sitomania', 'trophomania' or 'orthomania'. 'Sitomania' (from the Greek word 'sîtos' meaning 'food') can express some manic relationship with food (Nyman, 2002). Thus, 'sitomania' refers to a 'morbid obsession with food' or 'mania for eating' (Bender, 2009). In 'trophomania', the term 'trophé' means 'nourishment' or 'food'. In 'orthomania', there is a lack of food term (Nyman, 2002). The already launched term 'orthorexia' is well-known as a term related to the fixation on food.

In the author's opinion, the use of the term 'orthorexia' seems to be etymologically inaccurate because it does not focus on eating pathology per se or on healthy food preoccupation. Per definition, the word 'orthorexia' has been used because of obsessive preoccupation with healthy eating. So, how can the term meaning 'right appetite' indicate the 'pathological fixation on eating proper food'? From the etymological origin of 'orthorexia', an interest in eating right or eating healthily is not related to a problematic approach to food (Barrada & Roncero, 2018). If we consider that excessive focus on healthy eating (or increasingly obsessive concerns about a healthy diet) and concern about one's health are pathognomonic symptoms of orthorexia nervosa, we have to change the terminology to describe this phenomenon more accurately. There is other evidence justifying a need to update the term that more accurately describes this phenomenon. A bidimensional structure of the orthorexia was previously proposed (Barrada & Roncero, 2018). The conceptualisation of orthorexia was expanded to include both problematic and non-problematic aspects of healthy eating: 'healthy orthorexia' and 'orthorexia nervosa'. The first one represents a healthy interest in diet, which is independent of psychopathology (eating disorders, obsessive-compulsive disorder and negative affect) and even inversely associated with it. The second one refers to a pathological preoccupation with a healthy diet (Barrada & Roncero, 2018). The question remains open: how the same term 'orthorexia', meaning an interest in 'eating right', could indicate, on the one hand, healthy eating behaviour not associated with a problematic approach to food and, on the other hand, unhealthy eating behaviour associated with a problematic approach to food? If we intend to describe two different eating behaviours, we should use two terms with different etymologies. Health concerns and preoccupation with healthy eating appear fundamental in this phenomenon. Therefore, a new term for describing a pathological focus on healthy eating may consist of 'salūs' meaning 'health', 'sîtos' meaning 'food', and the suffix '-mania' meaning 'a very strong interest in something that fills a person's mind or uses up all their time' (Cambridge Dictionary). Thus, combining these three relevant elements may open the floodgates of the same concept with an etymologically distinct term called '*salussitomania*', literally meaning '*a very strong interest in health and food*'. Focusing on the original term 'orthorexia', the author would like to draw attention to the fact that there is a need to achieve a consensus on its adequate terminology. This may help to give accurate names to various phenomena and differentiate between healthy and pathological eating behaviours. *The launched term 'orthorexia nervosa' is well-known for its fixation on healthy eating and is widely used in the literature. Therefore, this term will be used within the existing findings and concepts in this book.*

From the therapeutic experience of the author, orthorexia nervosa is an outgrowth of health concerns. As a result of excessive focus on one's health, a person undertakes specific inappropriate eating behaviours, resulting in preoccupation with eating healthy food (Figure 3.1).

Thus, the dimensional structure of healthy eating could be conceptualised on a continuum from healthy relations with food to excessive preoccupation with healthy eating. It is worth pointing out that eating behaviour dimensions could influence food intake through choices about what, when and where to eat (Salmela et al., 2023).

The previous findings support a dimensional approach to eating pathology (Luo et al., 2016). Eating disorders have been proposed to be best conceptualised as dimensional in nature, in that eating pathology was distributed on a continuum within the population, and differences between various forms of eating pathology were quantitative in nature rather than qualitative. More

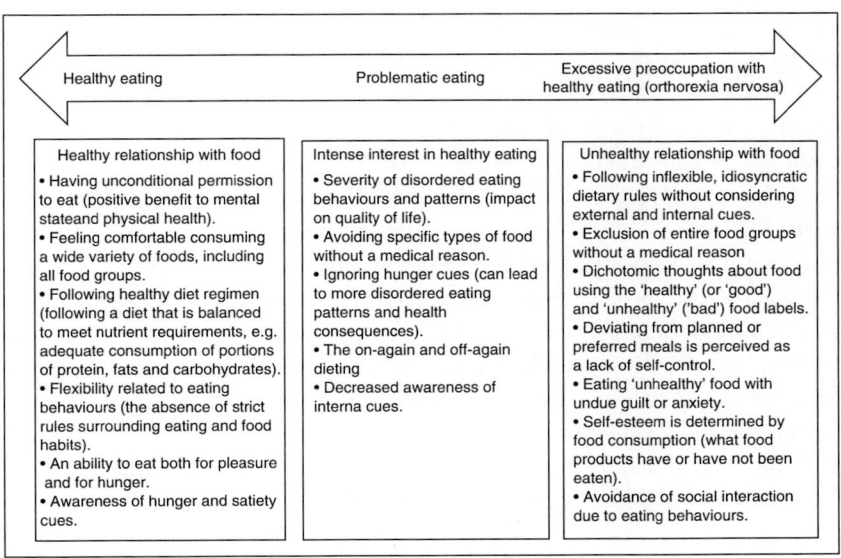

Figure 3.1 The continuum of healthy eating: taking healthy eating to an extreme.

precisely, the conceptualisation of eating pathology around its core dimensions (such as, e.g. body dissatisfaction and weight preoccupation) has been suggested instead of classifying eating pathology into various categorical diagnoses. An eating disorder diagnosis has been proposed to include severity specifications on each core dimension as well as a specification of related impairment. In this way, subclinical symptoms that are hard to classify can be better understood using a set of latent dimensions. Furthermore, the crossover of diagnoses could be understood as quantitative changes along dimensions instead of changes in the nature of the pathology or diagnosis (Luo et al., 2016). We can raise whether we may adopt a dimensional framework when considering orthorexia nervosa. Based on the previous research (Luo et al., 2016), it is worth considering whether a knowledge of the core dimension(s) of orthorexia nervosa (we could consider a preoccupation with healthy eating focused on the nutritional quality of the food and/or health preoccupation) and an awareness that individuals can have varying levels of severity on this (these) dimension(s) would allow the clinicians and researchers to provide a more nuanced understanding of pathology.

## 3.2 Global Study Distribution on Orthorexia Nervosa

The first study in the field was published in English two decades ago in Italy (Donini et al., 2004). Lorenzo Donini et al. (2004) aimed to propose a diagnosis of orthorexia nervosa and to verify its prevalence. The findings have reported that 6.9% of individuals (out of 404 taking part in the study) presented with orthorexia nervosa. The prevalence of orthorexia nervosa was higher in men and individuals with a lower level of education. The authors suggested that a protocol for diagnosis of orthorexia nervosa should be based on both the presence of a disorder with obsessive-compulsive personality features (measured by the psychasthenia subscale of the Minnesota Multiphasic Personality Inventory) and an exaggerated healthy eating behaviour pattern (measured by 'a questionnaire on eating behaviour which examines the quality, rather than the quantity', p. 155). The same year, Cartwright (2004) reviewed for the first time in English 'another disordered eating pattern, orthorexia nervosa' that 'has not been classified as a true eating disorder' and presented a clinical vignette of a 53-year-old man who suffered from orthorexia nervosa.

The number of papers on orthorexia nervosa has increased over the last two decades, with ever-growing numbers of publications from 2017 (Figure 3.2).

Research on orthorexia nervosa has been conducted across different continents (Figure 3.3).

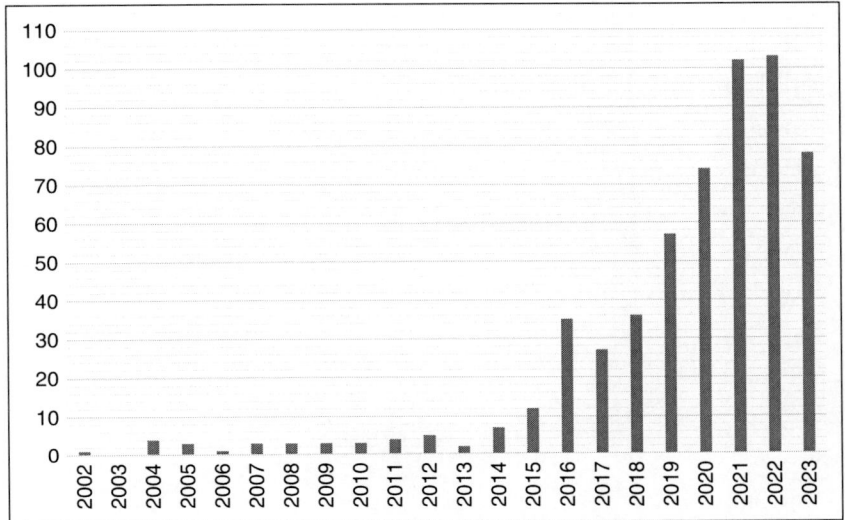

Figure 3.2 Number of PubMed articles with the term 'orthorexia' from 2002 to 2023.
Note: Stop data collection on 15 December 2023.

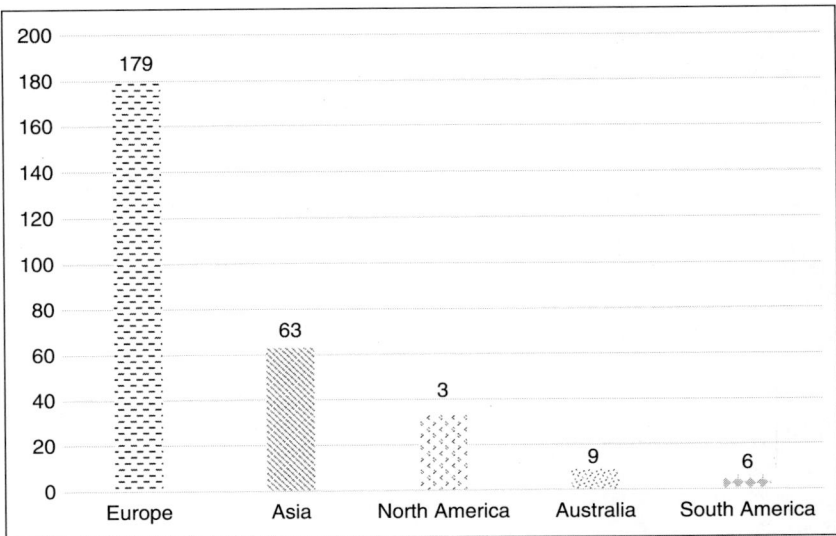

Figure 3.3 Published research findings on orthorexia nervosa in the studies reported in English across continents.
Note: Stop data collection on 1 July 2023.

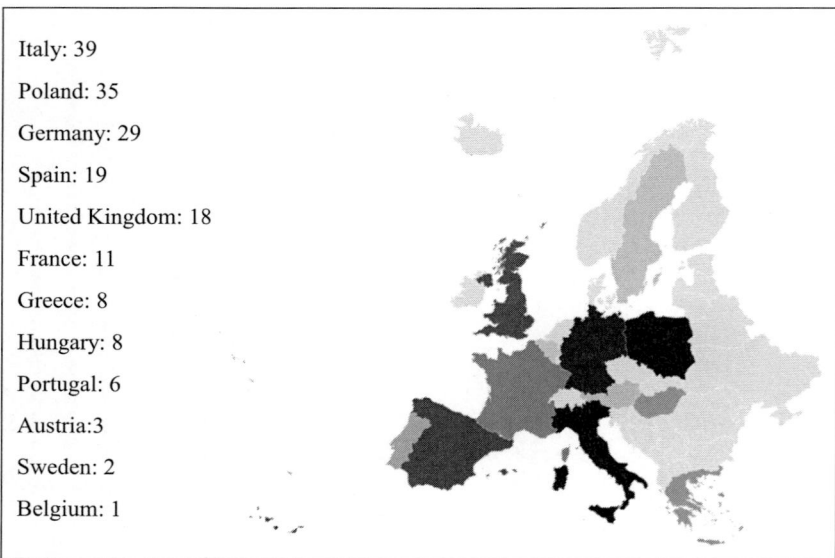

Italy: 39

Poland: 35

Germany: 29

Spain: 19

United Kingdom: 18

France: 11

Greece: 8

Hungary: 8

Portugal: 6

Austria:3

Sweden: 2

Belgium: 1

**Figure 3.4** Published research findings on orthorexia nervosa in the studies reported in English in Europe.
Note: Stop data collection on 1 July 2023.

The largest part of the studies has been conducted in Europe (61.05%), especially in Italy (22.41%) and in Poland (20.11%) (Figure 3.4).

Since 2007, more than 30 studies have been conducted in this field in Asian countries (22.11%), especially in Turkey (46.03%) and Lebanon (38.09%). Research has also been carried out in North America (11.58%), solely in the United States (69.70%) and Canada (30.30%). Relatively few studies have been performed in Australia (3.16%) and South America (2.10%), mainly in Brazil (83.33%).

# 4 Diagnostic Overview of Orthorexia Nervosa

Diagnosis is relevant for patient care, research and policy. When an accurate and 'timely' diagnosis is made, a patient has the best opportunity for a positive health outcome because clinical decision-making will be tailored to a correct understanding of the patient's health problem (Balogh et al., 2015). During the development of the 11th version of the International Statistical Classification of Diseases and Related Health Problems (ICD-11) and the 5th edition of the Diagnostic and Statistical Manual of Mental Disorders (DSM-5), the World Health Organization and the American Psychiatric Association (APA) made efforts towards harmonising the two classification systems: (1) for a more accurate collection of national health statistics and design of clinical trials aimed at developing new treatments, (2) to increase the ability to replicate scientific findings across national boundaries and (3) to rectify the issue of DSM-IV and ICD-10 diagnoses not agreeing (Bridley & Daffin, 2023).

At present, orthorexia nervosa is not officially recognised as a distinct disorder (an autonomous or additional eating disorder) in the DSM-5 or the ICD-11. According to the DSM Steering Committee (APA, 2021), a new diagnostic category included in the DSM-5 has to meet the criteria for a mental disorder, have strong evidence of validity or clinical utility, be capable of being applied reliably, manifest substantial clinical value, avoid substantial overlap with existing diagnoses or subtypes and have a positive benefit/harm ratio. In the DSM-5, the concept of dysfunction takes precedence (Telles-Correia, Saraiva & Gonçalves, 2018, p. 3):

*A mental disorder is a syndrome characterised by clinically significant disturbance in an individual's cognition, emotion regulation, or behaviour that reflects a dysfunction in the psychological, biological, or developmental processes underlying mental functioning. Mental disorders are usually associated with significant distress or disability in social, occupational, or other important activities.* (APA, 2013)

It is worth pointing out that mental disorders included in the DSM have a systematic observation of patterns of illness (including characteristic symptoms, course and outcomes among patients) (Surís et al., 2016) and are empirically based. For orthorexia nervosa, these conditions are not yet fulfilled. The existing literature does not permit researchers to provide strong evidence that orthorexia nervosa has diagnostic stability (Brytek-Matera, 2023).

According to Robins and Guze (1970), 'a valid classification is an essential step in science' (p. 107). The diagnostic schemes must be based on systematic studies rather than a priori principles. The authors have found that the five phases facilitate the development of a valid classification in psychiatry (originally, this phase was applied to schizophrenia) (Table 4.1). The authors (Robins & Guze, 1970) indicate that these five phases interact, so new findings in any of the phases may lead to modifications in one or more of the other phases.

To date, solely one of the five phases of the achievement of diagnostic validity for a mental disorder is wholly fulfilled, that is, a clinical description of orthorexia nervosa. A fully validated diagnostic classification of orthorexia nervosa still requires reliable laboratory studies as well as the exclusion of other disorders. There are no follow-up and family studies of orthorexia nervosa in the literature.

Nowadays, the main challenge is developing uniform diagnostic criteria based on research, clinical data and expert consensus. Following this, whether orthorexia nervosa should be based on an evidence-based diagnostic classification system, or perhaps whether a transdiagnostic approach should be considered, is a question worth pondering. More and more scientists are noticing that the usefulness of the current psychiatric classification, which is based on DSM-5 (or DSM-5-TR) or ICD-11 categorical diagnoses (gold standard) which demonstrate moderate to almost perfect reliability, remains questionable (Dalgleish et al., 2020; Fusar-Poli et al., 2019; Wakefield, 2016).

*Traditional diagnostic systems may no longer be fit for purpose for classifying mental ill health, facilitating understanding of its core underlying biopsychosocial processes, nor driving clinical developments. Here we propose that 'transdiagnostic' approaches have the potential to represent better the clinical and scientific reality of mental health problems, reflecting the complexity, dimensionality and comorbidity that is the norm in clinical practice.* (Dalgleish et al., 2020, p. 179)

Thus, some 'TRANSD' diagnostic guidelines have been proposed to improve the consistency and quality of the next generation of transdiagnostic research (Fusar-Poli et al., 2019, p. 203):

- Transparent definition of the gold standard (ICD, DSM), including specific diagnostic types, official codes, primary versus secondary diagnoses and diagnostic assessment interviews.
- Report the study's primary outcome, design and definition of the transdiagnostic construct in the abstract and main text.
- Appraise the conceptual framework/approach of the transdiagnostic approach: across-diagnoses, beyond-diagnoses, other.
- Numerate the diagnostic categories, spectra and non-clinical samples in which the transdiagnostic construct is being tested and then validated.
- Show the degree of improvement of the transdiagnostic approach against the specific diagnostic approach through specific comparative analyses.
- Demonstrate the generalisability of the transdiagnostic construct through external validation studies.

**Table 4.1** Five phases of method for achieving a high degree of diagnostic validity in mental disorder in the context of orthorexia nervosa

| Phase of the establishment of diagnostic validity for a mental disorder | Characteristics | Studies on orthorexia nervosa |
|---|---|---|
| Clinical description | • Description of the clinical picture of the disorder (e.g. a single striking clinical feature or a combination of clinical features). | There are research studies on this topic |
| Laboratory study | • Consistent and reliable laboratory findings, i.e. chemical, physiological, radiological and anatomical findings, as well as psychological tests showing reproducibility and reliability.<br><br>• When laboratory studies are consistent with a defined clinical picture, they permit a more refined classification. | • There is a lack of chemical, physiological, radiological and anatomical studies.<br><br>• Solely one neuropsychological study has been conducted so far (Koven & Senbonmatsu, 2013).<br><br>• Despite several existing methods (see Part III), no generally accepted tool(s) exists. |
| Exclusion of other disorders | • Since similar clinical features and laboratory findings may occur in patients suffering from different disorders, it is necessary to specify exclusion criteria to determine which patients should be included in the study group.<br><br>• These criteria should also permit the exclusion of borderline cases and doubtful cases so that the index group may be as homogeneous as possible. | • So far, there is no substantial evidence that orthorexia nervosa should be considered a distinct mental illness.<br><br>• Previous studies have demonstrated an overlap between orthorexia nervosa, and anorexia nervosa and obsessive-compulsive disorder (McComb & Mills, 2019).<br><br>• Two studies have demonstrated that clinical impairment, well-being, life satisfaction and chronic stress were no longer related to orthorexia nervosa when controlling for symptoms of eating disorder (Strahler et al., 2018; Zickgraf et al., 2019). |

Table 4.1 (cont.)

| Phase of the establishment of diagnostic validity for a mental disorder | Characteristics | Studies on orthorexia nervosa |
|---|---|---|
| Follow-up study | • Detecting if or not the original patients are suffering from some other defined disorder that could account for the original clinical picture.<br>• If patients are suffering from another such illness, this finding suggests that the original patients did not comprise a homogeneous group and that it is necessary to modify the diagnostic criteria.<br>• In the absence of known aetiology or pathogenesis, marked differences in outcome (such as between complete recovery and chronic illness) suggest that the group is not homogeneous. | Lack of research studies on the topic. |
| Family study | • Studying the hereditary or environmental causes.<br>• Assessment of the increased or decreased prevalence of the same disorder among the patients' close relatives. | Lack of research studies on the topic. |

Source: Based on Robins and Guze (1970).

## 4.1 Review of Existing Diagnostic Criteria

The four sets of classification criteria for orthorexia nervosa have been developed so far (Table 4.2). The first of them was proposed by Setnick in 2013, less than 16 years after the description of orthorexia nervosa (Bratman, 1997). The last classification criteria for orthorexia nervosa were proposed by Dunn and Bratman in 2016.

The four sets of diagnostic criteria of orthorexia nervosa have three common features: (1) a pathological preoccupation with healthy eating; (2) psychological and medical consequences (e.g. clinically relevant distress with feelings of guilt, shame, anxiety, disability in important areas of life, significant weight loss, malnutrition); and (3) eating disturbance is not attributable to another mental disorder such as anorexia nervosa or obsessive-compulsive disorder (Brytek-Matera, 2023). It is worth adding that validation studies should be sought to confirm the proposed criteria.

To date, there is still a lack of a gold standard for diagnosis and universally agreed upon diagnostic criteria for orthorexia nervosa (Brytek-Matera, 2023). Therefore, an international, multidisciplinary group of experts (Orthorexia Nervosa Task Force; ON-TF) has been working on determining diagnostic criteria for orthorexia nervosa for a few years (Cena et al., 2019; Donini et al., 2022). In 2019, the Orthorexia Nervosa Task Force (Cena et al., 2019) summarised three primary diagnostic criteria for orthorexia nervosa: (1) a pathological preoccupation with healthy eating; (2) the emotional consequences (e.g. stress or anxiety) of non-compliance with self-imposed dietary rules; and (3) psychosocial impairments in significant areas of life, malnutrition and weight loss. Donini and colleagues (2022) have recently proposed tentative diagnostic criteria within the Orthorexia Nervosa Task Force framework. Criterion A is focused on the definition, clinical aspects and duration of orthorexia nervosa. Criterion B is related to the consequences of orthorexia nervosa. Criterion C involves the onset of orthorexia nervosa, whereas criterion D refers to the exclusion criteria of orthorexia nervosa (Donini et al., 2022). The 27 proposed criteria concerning orthorexia nervosa and its related risk factors (e.g. a history of eating disorders or mental disorders), pathophysiology (e.g. nutritional deficiencies, hormonal disturbances), clinical, psychological and functional consequences can be used as agreed upon criteria for screening research participants, evaluating treatment protocols, and expanding prevalence data between groups (Donini et al., 2022). There is no doubt that by specifying reliable criteria in the foreseeable future, the proper diagnosis of orthorexia nervosa could be made in both clinical and non-clinical samples.

Table 4.2 Existing diagnostic criteria for orthorexia nervosa

| Criterion | Setnick, 2013 | Moroze et al., 2015 | Barthels et al., 2015a | Dunn and Bratman, 2016 |
|---|---|---|---|---|
| A | Pathological preoccupation with nutrition and diet far beyond that which is necessary for health and undue influence of diet on self-evaluation, evidenced by characteristics such as:<br><br>A1. Phobic avoidance of or response to foods perceived to be unhealthy;<br><br>A2. Severe emotional distress or self-harm after eating a food considered unhealthy;<br><br>A3. Persistent failure to meet appropriate nutritional needs leading to nutritional deficit and/or psychological dependence on individual nutrient supplements in place of food intake due to the belief | Obsessional preoccupation with eating 'healthy foods', focusing on concerns regarding the quality and composition of meals.<br><br>At least two or more of the following:<br><br>A1. Consuming a nutritionally unbalanced diet due to preoccupying beliefs about food 'purity';<br><br>A2. Preoccupation and worries about eating impure or unhealthy foods and the impact of food quality and composition on physical and/ or emotional health;<br><br>A3. Rigid avoidance of foods believed by the patient to be 'unhealthy'; | Enduring and intensive preoccupation with healthy nutrition, healthy foods and healthy eating. | Obsessive focus on 'healthy' eating marked by exaggerated emotional distress in relationship to food choices perceived as unhealthy.<br><br>As evidenced by the following:<br><br>A1. Compulsive behaviour and/or mental preoccupation regarding affirmative and restrictive dietary practices believed by the individual to promote optimum health.<br><br>A2. Violation of self-imposed dietary rules causes exaggerated fear of disease, a sense of personal impurity and/or negative physical sensations accompanied by anxiety and shame. |

Table 4.2 (Cont. – Part A)

| Criterion | Setnick, 2013 | Moroze et al., 2015 | Barthels et al., 2015a | Dunn and Bratman, 2016 |
|---|---|---|---|---|
| | that synthetic nutrients are superior to those found in food or that food is contaminated; | A4. Excessive amounts of time spent reading about, acquiring and/or preparing specific types of foods based on their perceived quality and composition; | | A3. Dietary restrictions escalate over time and may include eliminating entire food groups and involve progressively more frequent and/or severe 'cleanses' regarded as purifying or detoxifying. This escalation commonly leads to weight loss, but the desire to lose weight is absent, hidden or subordinated to ideation about healthy eating. |
| | A4. Following a restrictive diet prescribed for a medical condition that the individual does not have or to prevent illness not known to be influenced by diet; | A5. Guilty feelings and worries after transgressions in which 'unhealthy' or 'impure' foods are consumed; | | |
| | A5. Insisting on the health benefits of the diet in the face of evidence to the contrary; | A6. Intolerance of others' food beliefs; | | |
| | A6. Marked interference with social functioning or activities of daily living, such as isolation when eating. | A7. Spending excessive amounts of money relative to one's income on foods because of their perceived quality and composition. | | |

Table 4.2 (Cont. – Part B)

| Criterion | Setnick, 2013 | Moroze et al., 2015 | Barthels et al., 2015a | Dunn and Bratman, 2016 |
|---|---|---|---|---|
| B | Not the result of a lack of available food or a culturally sanctioned practice. | Obsessional preoccupation becomes impairing by either of the following: **B1**. Impairment of physical health owing to nutritional imbalances; **B2**. Severe distress or impairment of social, academic or vocational functioning owing to obsessional thoughts and behaviours focusing on the patient's beliefs about 'healthy' eating. | Anxieties and extensive avoidance of foods considered unhealthy according to subjective beliefs. | Compulsive behaviour and mental preoccupation become clinically impairing by any of the following: **B1**. Malnutrition, severe weight loss or other medical complications from restricted diet. **B2**. Intrapersonal distress or impairment of social, academic or vocational functioning secondary to beliefs or behaviours about healthy diet. **B3**. Positive body image, self-worth, identity and/or satisfaction depend excessively on compliance with self-defined 'healthy' eating behaviour. |

Table 4.2 (Cont. – Part C)

| Criterion | Setnick, 2013 | Moroze et al., 2015 | Barthels et al., 2015a | Dunn and Bratman, 2016 |
|---|---|---|---|---|
| C | Individual endorses a drive for health or life extension rather than a drive for thinness. | Disturbance is not merely an exacerbation of the symptoms of another disorder. | **C1.** At least two overvalued ideas concerning the effectiveness and potential health benefits of foods and/ or<br><br>**C2.** Ritualised preoccupation with buying, preparing and consuming foods is not due to culinary reasons but stems from overvalued ideas. Deviation or impossibility of adhering to nutrition rules causes intensive fears, which can be avoided by a rigid adherence to the rules. | - |

Table 4.2 (Cont. – Part D)

| Criterion | Setnick, 2013 | Moroze et al., 2015 | Barthels et al., 2015a | Dunn and Bratman, 2016 |
|---|---|---|---|---|
| D | Eating disturbance is not attributable to a medical condition or another mental disorder. | Behaviour is not better accounted for by the exclusive observation of organised orthodox religious food observance or when concerns with specialised food requirements are in relation to professionally diagnosed food allergies or medical conditions requiring a specific diet. | **D1.** The fixation on healthy eating causes suffering or impairments of clinical relevance in social, occupational or other important areas of life and/ or negatively affects children and/or<br><br>**D2.** Deficiency syndrome due to disordered eating behaviour. Insight into the illness is not necessary; in some cases, the lack of insight might be an indicator of the severity of the disorder. | - |
| E | - | - | Intended weight loss and underweight may be present, but worries about weight and shape should not dominate the syndrome. | - |

Source: Based on Brytek-Matera (2023).

# 5 Orthorexia Nervosa and Other Disorders: Differential Diagnosis

Is orthorexia nervosa a healthy way of being or a mental health disorder? Classification of orthorexia nervosa is currently being debated. Up to now, orthorexia nervosa has been regarded as a new mental illness (Koven & Abry, 2015), a lifestyle phenomenon (Håman et al., 2015) or a behavioural pattern (Strahler et al., 2018). In a little more than a decade, the author wondered what kind of disorder orthorexia nervosa is (Brytek-Matera, 2012). It has been indicated that:

*Orthorexia nervosa could not be labelled as a new eating disorder because it does not include the most characteristic symptoms of anorexia and bulimia nervosa, that is, immense fear of becoming fat, extreme weight-control behaviour as well as overvaluation of shape and weight. However, since orthorexia involves disturbance of eating habits, it ought to be treated as a disorder concerning abnormal eating behaviour inseparably linked with obsessive-compulsive symptoms (on account of paying too much attention to consuming healthy food and constant thinking about the quality of food intake)* (p. 59).

Despite the passage of time, no clear consensus has yet emerged as to whether orthorexia nervosa should be considered (1) as a diagnostic entity that is distinct from established eating disorders and obsessive-compulsive disorder, (2) on the eating disorder spectrum or (3) on the obsessive-compulsive spectrum. Some researchers postulate that orthorexia nervosa should be regarded as a separate eating disorder category (Cosh et al., 2023; Zickgraf et al., 2019), as the moderate effect size observed indicates that orthorexia nervosa and anorexia nervosa are related but still distinct (Zickgraf et al., 2019). While other researchers disagree with the statement that orthorexia nervosa represents a distinct diagnostic entity (associations of orthorexia nervosa with a core of symptoms of eating disorders question the potential of orthorexia nervosa as a distinct diagnosis; Hessler-Kaufmann et al., 2021) and suggest that orthorexia nervosa may instead be an aspect of restrictive eating disorder symptomatology (Meule & Voderholzer, 2021) or a subclinical and asymptomatic form of an eating disorder (Strahler et al., 2018) or a distinct subtype of avoidant/restrictive food intake disorder (Dell'Osso et al., 2016; Moroze et al., 2015) or a new cultural manifestation of anorexia nervosa caused by modern-day diet culture and healthism (Bhattacharya et al., 2022). However, the previous systematic review of the literature (Atchison & Zickgraf, 2022) has indicated that orthorexia nervosa is consistently related to both trait and disordered restrictive eating symptoms of anorexia nervosa and weight control motivations for food choice. The finding that orthorexia nervosa is related to restraint and weight loss efforts but not to body dissatisfaction or dysregulated eating suggests that orthorexia nervosa may represent a distinct eating disorder (Atchison & Zickgraf, 2022).

## 5.1 Comparison between Orthorexia Nervosa and Anorexia Nervosa: Similarities and Differences

Two questions remain open: (1) Should orthorexia be considered a special diagnostic category? and (2) whether the symptoms of orthorexia nervosa could be a manifestation of another, clinically recognised eating disorder, namely anorexia nervosa? (Table 5.1).

A recent systematic review and meta-analysis (Zagaria et al., 2022) have revealed that orthorexia nervosa shares overlap with several existing disorders. Orthorexia nervosa and anorexia nervosa share similar clinical presentations (Table 5.2).

However, the main difference between orthorexia nervosa and anorexia nervosa concerns the reason for food refusal: in orthorexia nervosa, food choices are based on qualitative, health-related aspects of foods for being healthy, whereas in anorexia nervosa, food choices are based on quantitative, energy density-related aspects of foods for creating weight loss (Cena et al., 2019). A preoccupation with weight loss, an intense fear of gaining weight, an excessive influence of shape and weight on self-evaluation and body image disturbances, which are crucial characteristics within the development and maintenance of anorexia nervosa, are not part of the proposed diagnostic criteria for orthorexia nervosa (Brytek-Matera et al., 2015a). Also, compensatory behaviour (binge eating and purging), which

Table 5.1 DSM-5 criteria for anorexia nervosa

| Criterion | Characteristics of diagnostic criteria |
| --- | --- |
| A | Restricting energy intake relative to requirements leads to a significantly low body weight in the context of age, sex, developmental trajectory and physical health. |
| B | Intense fear of gaining weight or becoming fat or persistent behaviour that interferes with weight gain, even though underweight. |
| C | Disturbance in the way in which one's body weight or shape is experienced, undue influence of body weight or shape on self-evaluation, or persistent lack of recognition of the seriousness of the current low body weight. |

Source: The Diagnostic and Statistical Manual of Mental Disorders, Fifth Edition (DSM-5), American Psychiatric Association (APA, 2013).

Table 5.2 Orthorexia nervosa and anorexia nervosa: similarities

Signs and symptoms common to orthorexia nervosa and anorexia nervosa
- Concern over food and eating
- Restrictive eating patterns and behaviours
- Excessive focus on food-related topics
- Adherence to diet as a marker of self-discipline
- Making eating-related issues the primary focus of one's own life
- Sense of superiority over others based on one's eating practices
- Self-realisation through the control of food intake
- Strict behaviour and rituals related to the preparation of food
- Intrusive food-related thoughts
- Intense anxiety regarding certain foods and their avoidance
- Intense fear of longer-term outcomes of eating fear foods
- Failure to follow a diet results in anxiety, guilt and shame
- Impairments in psychosocial functioning (e.g. social isolation)
- Obsessive-compulsive personality traits (e.g. perfectionism, rigidity)
- Ego-syntonicity of symptoms
- Malnutrition

Source: Based on Brytek-Matera (2023).

is a crucial characteristic of binge eating/purging type of anorexia nervosa, is not part of the proposed diagnostic criteria for orthorexia nervosa (binge eating/ purging type of anorexia nervosa according to the DSM-5) (Brytek-Matera, 2023). Contradictory findings have indicated female predominance or male predominance or no sex differences in orthorexia nervosa (Brytek-Matera, 2023), while the epidemiological study has revealed the predominance of anorexia nervosa in women (van Eeden, van Hoeken & Hoek, 2021).

The findings have demonstrated that the increased prevalence of symptoms of orthorexia nervosa is significantly associated with high rates of symptoms of eating disorders (Zagaria et al., 2022). It is worth pointing out that eating disorders have been identified as risk factors for orthorexia nervosa (Segura-Garcia et al., 2015) or negative predictors of orthorexia nervosa (Barrada & Roncero, 2018). It has been proposed that orthorexia nervosa may precede the onset of anorexia nervosa (and thus represents a prodromal phase of eating difficulties; Segura-Garcia et al., 2015) or follow its onset (Cartwright, 2004) or represent its evolution in the phase of remission and recovery (Segura-Garcia et al., 2015; Gramaglia et al., 2019). Orthorexia nervosa may represent a socially approved way to express symptoms of anorexia nervosa (Brytek-Matera et al., 2015b) and thus may be conceived as an efficient attempt to maintain certain ego-syntonic and dysfunctional eating habits (Shah, 2012). Focusing on healthy eating is socially acceptable; nevertheless, it is worth remembering that orthorexic behaviour can hide the real attempt to control the amount of food intake with the excuse of consuming high-quality foods (Segura-Garcia et al., 2015).

## 5.2 Comparison between Orthorexia Nervosa and Obsessive-Compulsive Disorder: Similarities and Differences

Several previous and recent studies (e.g. Costa et al., 2019; Hallit et al., 2022; Novara et al., 2021; Mahfoud et al., 2023; Vaccari et al., 2021; more references are disponible in the recent reviews and meta-analyses by Zagaria et al., 2022 and by Huynh et al., 2023) have investigated the relationship between orthorexia nervosa and obsessive-compulsive disorder (Table 5.3).

There is initial evidence confirming the similar behavioural and thinking patterns in orthorexia nervosa and obsessive-compulsive disorder (Brytek-Matera et al., 2017, 2022; Cena et al., 2019; Koven & Abry, 2015) (Table 5.4).

Table 5.3 DSM-5 criteria for obsessive-compulsive disorder

| Criterion | Characteristics of diagnostic criteria |
| --- | --- |
| A | Presence of obsessions, compulsions, or both:<br><br>*Obsessions* are defined by (1) and (2):<br>(1) Recurrent and persistent thoughts, urges or impulses that are experienced, at some time during the disturbance, as intrusive and unwanted and that in most individuals cause marked anxiety or distress.<br>(2) The individual attempts to ignore or suppress such thoughts, urges or images or to neutralise them with some other thought or action (i.e. by performing a compulsion).<br><br>*Compulsions* are defined by (1) and (2):<br>(1) Repetitive behaviours (e.g. hand washing, ordering, checking) or mental acts (e.g. praying, counting, repeating words silently) that the individual feels driven to perform in response to an obsession or according to rules that must be applied rigidly.<br>(2) The behaviours or mental acts are aimed at preventing or reducing distress or preventing some dreaded event or situation; however, these behaviours or mental acts are not connected in a realistic way with what they are designed to neutralise or prevent or are excessive. |
| B | The obsessions or compulsions are time-consuming (e.g. take more than one hour per day) or cause clinically significant distress or impairment in social, occupational or other important areas of functioning. |

Table 5.3 (cont.)

| Criterion | Characteristics of diagnostic criteria |
|---|---|
| C | The obsessive-compulsive symptoms are not attributable to the physiological effects of a substance (e.g. a drug of abuse, a medication) or another medical condition. |
| D | The disturbance is not better explained by the symptoms of another mental disorder (e.g. excessive worries, as in generalised anxiety disorder; preoccupation with appearance, as in body dysmorphic disorder; difficulty discarding or parting with possessions, as in hoarding disorder; hair pulling, as in trichotillomania [hair pulling disorder]; skin picking, as in excoriation [skin picking] disorder; stereotypies, as in stereotypic movement disorder; ritualised eating behaviour, as in eating disorders; preoccupation with substances or gambling, as in substance-related and addictive disorders; preoccupation with having an illness, as in illness anxiety disorder; sexual urges or fantasies, as in paraphilic disorders; impulses, as in disruptive, impulse-control and conduct disorders; guilty ruminations, as in major depressive disorder; thought insertion or delusional preoccupations, as in schizophrenia spectrum and other psychotic disorders; or repetitive patterns of behaviour, as in autism spectrum disorder). |

Source: The Diagnostic and Statistical Manual of Mental Disorders, Fifth Edition (DSM-5), American Psychiatric Association (APA, 2013).

## Table 5.4 Overlapping behavioural and cognitive characteristics of orthorexia nervosa and obsessive-compulsive disorder

Signs and symptoms common to orthorexia nervosa and obsessive-compulsive disorder
- Recurrent, intrusive thoughts (e.g. on planning meals)
- Repeating behaviours (e.g. ritualised patterns of food preparation with a tendency to spend an unusual amount of time managing food and planning meals)
- Cognitive inflexibility
- Perfectionism
- Impairment in psychosocial function (e.g. social isolation)
- Need to exert control
- Perfectionism
- High anxiety traits (e.g. about contaminated food)
- Depression
- Feeling guilty (e.g. poor adherence to one's own rules for healthy eating)
- Concerns about contamination

Source: Based on Brytek-Matera et al. (2022).

Despite the existing similarities, the main discrepancy between orthorexia nervosa and obsessive-compulsive disorder stems from their different nature: the nature of egosyntonicity in orthorexia nervosa and the nature of egodystonicity in obsessive-compulsive disorder (Mathieu, 2005). Moreover, the obsessive-compulsive symptoms found in individuals with orthorexia nervosa may be uniquely linked with food preoccupation and not with full-blown obsessive-compulsive disorder (Costanzo et al., 2022).

Some evidence has indicated that individuals with orthorexia nervosa are more likely to report higher symptoms of obsessive-compulsive disorder (McComb & Mills, 2019). Previous findings (Brytek-Matera et al., 2022) demonstrated that orthorexia nervosa is partially independent of obsessive-compulsive disorder in the non-clinical sample. At the same time, other results suggested high comorbidity between the two conditions (Duradoni et al., 2023). There are also studies (Bartel et al., 2020) revealing that orthorexia nervosa is less related to obsessive-compulsive disorder than to eating disorders. Orthorexic symptoms seem to be distinct from obsessive-compulsive disorder. In addition, the low effect size observed for the relationship between these two conditions may be interpreted as evidence that orthorexia nervosa and obsessive-compulsive disorder are two separate disorders (Zagaria et al., 2022). In contrast, the findings of the recent systematic review and meta-analysis (Huynh et al., 2023) demonstrated a relationship between orthorexia nervosa and obsessive-compulsive symptoms. Thirty-three (out of 40) studies reported at least one significant association between orthorexia nervosa and obsessive-compulsive symptoms, with correlation strength varying from negligible to large: 17 studies found at least 1 small but significant correlation, 14 studies found moderate correlations and 2 studies found a large correlation, while 7 studies found no significant correlation (Huynh et al., 2023).

The presence of symptoms of obsessive-compulsive disorder in individuals with orthorexia nervosa may be due to the overlap between orthorexia nervosa and anorexia nervosa and, consequently, to the high rates of comorbidity between anorexia nervosa and obsessive-compulsive disorder (Costanzo et al., 2022). It has also been proposed that orthorexia nervosa could evolve into obsessive-compulsive symptomatology at some points in the eating disorder course (Costa & Hardan-Khalil, 2019). In this case, orthorexia nervosa can be regarded as a combination of anorexia nervosa and obsessive-compulsive disorder because it shares several characteristics of both diseases (Costa & Hardan-Khalil, 2019). Neurocognitive deficits, including impairments in flexible problem-solving, external attention and working memory, have been identified in patients with these conditions (Koven & Abry, 2013; Koven & Senbonmatsu, 2013). Possible biochemical similarities have been found that can influence thought patterns and behaviours in both orthorexia nervosa and obsessive-compulsive disorder (Costa & Hardan-Khalil, 2019). Patients with obsessive-compulsive disorder and eating disorders have higher cerebral glucose metabolism, which does not allow them to effectively complete a task that requires the work of the prefrontal cortex and caudate nucleus of the brain (Murphy et al., 2004). Similar neurophysiological similarities have been implied in orthorexia nervosa and obsessive-compulsive disorder (Murphy et al., 2004).

### 5.2.1 Expert Commentary: Thoughts on Orthorexia Nervosa and Obsessive-Compulsive Disorder
by Caterina Novara, PhD

**Caterina Novara**, PhD is Associate Professor and Head of the Cognitive and Behavioral Therapy Service and postgraduate specialisation in clinical psychology in the Department of General Psychology at the University of Padova. She has published a number of peer-reviewed articles and book chapters related to her work on cognition, behaviour, anxiety and disordered eating, and is an invited speaker at national and international conferences. She is a fellow of the Italian Association of Psychology (AIP), Italian Association of Analysis and Behavior Modification (AIAMC) and European Association of Behavioral and Cognitive Therapy (EABCT).

Affiliation: Department of General Psychology, University of Padova, Italy.

Since its first introduction orthorexia nervosa has been defined in terms of excessive concern or obsession with healthy or pure foods and a lifestyle in line with this regimen (Bratman, 1997; Bratman & Knight, 2000). These observations acquire relevance following the study conducted by Donini et al. (2004), in which orthorexia nervosa is defined as 'an obsession' for healthy food, unlike anorexia and bulimia nervosa, whose psychopathological nucleus regards the amount of food. The authors highlight how the purity of food is highly relevant for individuals in this condition, even more than the physical damage resulting from an unbalanced diet. The lack of consensus about orthorexia nervosa as an independent disorder or a new syndrome related to eating disorders and/ or to obsessive-compulsive disorder spectrum (i.e. Cheshire, Berry & Fixsen, 2020) led groups of experts (i.e. Donini et al., 2022) to the definition of some characteristics of orthorexia nervosa as disordered eating with an exaggerated focus on the quality of food in order to control dietary habits in a healthy way (Yakin et al., 2022). In addition, orthorexia nervosa would be characterised by over-concerns or obsessions about food that interfere with everyday functioning; most problems would include pervasive preoccupation with food, a great amount of time spent preparing meals or selecting/checking food for its nutritional or purity components. Moreover, people with orthorexic symptomatology would have high levels of distress when their meals do not align with their beliefs about healthy eating.

According to a recent review (Cena et al., 2019), some of the core themes of orthorexia nervosa are similar to the broad range of eating disorders: the substantial concerns about food, the crucial role of eating in one's life, and the strong beliefs about a proper diet. In these respect, orthorexia nervosa is most often compared to anorexia nervosa, with which it shares dietary restriction, body dissatisfaction, an ideal of thinness and perfectionistic traits (Brytek-Matera et al., 2015a; Chaki et al., 2013; Koven & Abry, 2013; Novara et al., 2022a). On the contrary, orthorexia nervosa seems to differ from eating disorders in focusing on food quality rather than quantity (Cena et al., 2019). While patients with anorexia nervosa and bulimia nervosa engage in food restriction, the main focus in orthorexia nervosa is food purity (Dunn & Bratman, 2016; Scarff, 2017). Also, in a more recent meta-analysis conducted by Zagaria et al. (2022), an attempt was made to clarify the extent of the relationship between orthorexic characteristics and eating disorders or obsessive-compulsive disorder symptoms. Confirming previous results, the study highlighted the strong association between orthorexia nervosa and the presence of eating disorder symptoms. In addition, a weak relationship between the symptomatology of the obsessive-compulsive and orthorexic features has been highlighted. Moreover, in a prospective study of a large non-clinical population, it was found that problematic orthorexic behaviours were related to the frequency of lifelong diets and with a past diagnosis of anorexia nervosa, while after six months, the tendency to thinness was the only construct that explained the orthorexic problematic behaviours. Furthermore, no obsessive-compulsive construct entered the study models (Novara et al., 2022b). This evidence supports the presence of nuclear factors combining orthorexia nervosa and eating disorders, showing that these conditions are very similar in the processes of onset and maintenance and their broader contents.

Eating disorders and especially anorexia nervosa are often in comorbidity with obsessive-compulsive disorder: anorexia nervosa was found in 10% of female obsessive-compulsive disorder cases, and obsessive-compulsive disorder was detected in 35–44% of anorexia nervosa cases (LaSalle et al., 2004; Pinto et al., 2006). Recent molecular and genetic studies have shown common genetic factors linking obsessive-compulsive disorder and anorexia nervosa (Lee, Hoppenbrouwers & Franken, 2019; Yilmaz et al., 2020). In addition, symptomatological features and obsessive-compulsive personality traits are considered risk factors in the development of eating disorders (Micali et al., 2017; Thornton & Russell, 1997). Compulsivity can be considered the epiphenomenon that characterises the association between eating disorders and obsessive-compulsive disorder. When defined in broad terms as the tendency to perform repetitive, unwanted, inflexible acts (i.e. Fineberg et al., 2016), it may concern a wide range of human behaviours, including obsessive-compulsive compulsions such as checking or eating disorder behaviours related to purging. When considering the functional specificity of each disorder, the model can be broader in considering the purpose and, therefore, the ritualised compulsivity in obsessive-compulsive disorder aimed at reducing anxiety or aimed at reducing body weight in eating disorders. Both behaviours reduce negative affect or anxiety, but intrusive thoughts shown by both psychopathological configurations (Belloch, Roncero & Perpina, 2016) are not always negatively evaluated by patients with eating disorders.

In a recent network analysis by Meier et al. (2020), the authors investigated the presence of obsessive-compulsive symptoms in individuals admitted for eating disorders (anorexia nervosa, bulimia nervosa and binge eating). The results showed that the importance of intrusive cognitions and the reduced control over them are relevant constructs in both disorders, without revealing symptom bridges between the two clusters of symptoms and confirming a symptomatological independence. In a subsequent network analysis (Vanzhula, Kinkel-Ram & Levinson, 2021), it was highlighted that only perfectionism is a bridging factor between obsessive-compulsive disorder and eating disorders, suggesting that it may explain the comorbidity and maintenance of both disorders. Therefore, these disorders may share a vulnerability attributable to transdiagnostic factors rather than exclusively to cognitive and behavioural symptoms directly related to eating disorders and obsessive-compulsive disorder. A positive association between maladaptive perfectionism and greater tendencies of orthorexia nervosa has been shown in different studies (Hayes et al., 2017; Novara et al., 2023; Oberle, Samaghabadi & Hughes, 2017; Parra-Fernández et al., 2018a). Similarly, a study conducted to investigate whether orthorexia was a different condition from obsessive-compulsive disorder or eating disorders has shown that there were relationships between orthorexia nervosa, eating disorders and maladaptive perfectionism regardless of the presence of obsessive-compulsive symptoms (Novara et al., 2021b, 2023). Moreover, overlaps with the perfectionism dimensions were often found in populations with obsessive-compulsive features or eating disorders (i.e. Limburg et al., 2017). Furthermore, concern over mistakes – considered a maladaptive aspect of perfectionism – was found to be the factor that best explained the compulsive characteristics in a sample of anorexic patients and resulted independent of recovery status (Levinson et al., 2018). High perfectionist standards often take the form of self-imposed rules. Some examples are not eating a particular food in patients with eating disorders and following a certain ritual to avoid contamination in obsessive-compulsive disorder. Consistent with Fairburn's transdiagnostic model of eating disorders (Fairburn, 2008), self-imposed standards of perfection are objectively excessive and debilitating. Indeed, they can have emotional, social, physical, cognitive and/or behavioural consequences. Despite this, they are tolerated because the self-evaluation depends on the pursuit and achievement of their goal. Moreover, these consequences may not be seen by the individual as adverse, as they are often interpreted as evidence that reaching the standard requires effort. In fact, very often, if the standard is easily reached, its level of difficulty is raised with the belief that the former was too low. Although the standards of perfection characterise eating disorders and the obsessive-compulsive disorder configuration (Shafran, Cooper & Fairburn, 2002), they require further studies in orthorexia nervosa. Future research may also consider other constructs. Intolerance of uncertainty is considered a transdiagnostic construct that can independently contribute to a number of psychological disorders, including eating disorders and obsessive-compulsive disorder (Knowles & Olatunji, 2023; Williams & Levinson, 2021). The basic psychopathology of eating disorders could be considered a maladaptive attempt to regain certainty about the events of life and consequently increase the sense of safety and familiarity (Sternheim, Startup & Schimdt, 2011). In patients with obsessive-compulsive disorder, compulsions could act as reassurances to reduce uncertainty and the perception of 'threat' regarding a possible damage while decreasing perceived personal responsibility (Kobori et al., 2012).

The sense of control also plays a central role in the aetiology and maintenance of various disorders. In particular, it has been observed that individuals who suffer from eating disorders deploy ritual behaviours of control over weight and physical fitness to assess their self-control, from which derives their self-esteem (Fairburn et al., 1999). In addition, it seems to explain the aetiology and maintenance of obsessive-compulsive disorder. The fear of losing control, in some cases, may explain the discrepancy between the sense of control and the desire for control present in patients with obsessive-compulsive disorder (Radomsky, 2022; Reuven-Magril et al., 2008). Overall, these constructs require further studies to identify effective intervention protocols to reduce orthorexic problems when focused on commonly shared aspects with obsessive-compulsive disorder and eating disorders such as perfectionism, tolerance of uncertainty or a sense of control.

## 5.3 Comparison between Orthorexia Nervosa and Avoidant/Restrictive Food Intake Disorder: Similarities and Differences

Almost a decade ago, it was proposed (Moroze et al., 2015) that orthorexia nervosa be classified as a distinct subtype of a new (DSM-5) eating disorder – Avoidant/Restrictive Food Intake Disorder (previously referred to as 'Selective Eating Disorder') (Table 5.5).

Concern over food and eating a rigid and narrow diet (Zickgraf, Ellis & Essayli, 2019), food avoidance and restriction due to fear of immediate

### Table 5.5 DSM-5 criteria for avoidant/restrictive food intake disorder

| Criterion | Characteristics of diagnostic criteria |
|---|---|
| A | An eating or feeding disturbance (e.g. apparent lack of interest in eating or food; avoidance based on the sensory characteristics of food; concern about aversive consequences of eating) as manifested by persistent failure to meet appropriate nutritional and/or energy needs associated with one (or more) of the following: <br> 1. Significant weight loss (or failure to achieve expected weight gain or faltering growth in children). <br> 2. Significant nutritional deficiency. <br> 3. Dependence on enteral feeding or oral nutritional supplements. <br> 4. Marked interference with psychosocial functioning. |
| B | The disturbance is not better explained by a lack of available food or by an associated culturally sanctioned practice. |
| C | The eating disturbance does not occur exclusively during the course of anorexia nervosa or bulimia nervosa, and there is no evidence of a disturbance in the way in which one's body weight or shape is experienced. |
| D | The eating disturbance is not attributable to a concurrent medical condition or not better explained by another mental disorder. When the eating disturbance occurs in the context of another mental disorder, the severity of the eating disturbance exceeds that routinely associated with the condition or disorder and warrants additional clinical attention. |

Source: The Diagnostic and Statistical Manual of Mental Disorders, Fifth Edition (DSM-5), American Psychiatric Association (APA, 2013).

consequences of eating (Huynh et al., 2023) and psychosocial impairment are common symptoms for these two conditions.

In contrast, the core diagnostic symptoms of avoidant-restrictive food intake disorder, low body weight and nutritional deficiencies (malnutrition) due to food restriction are distinct from symptoms of orthorexia nervosa. In orthorexia nervosa, food restriction is the result of worries about the healthiness of a certain food, and malnutrition may represent a consequence of orthorexia nervosa and not a diagnostic marker (Donini et al., 2022). The avoidance of food, mainly occurring in (early) childhood and typically due to sensory characteristics of qualities of foods (e.g. smell, colour, texture), concern about the aversive consequences of eating, apparent lack of interest in eating and selective eating (Donini et al., 2022; Zickgraf, Ellis & Essayli, 2019) in avoidant/restrictive food intake disorder is not representative per se for orthorexia nervosa (Dunn & Bratman, 2016). Additionally, long-term health consequences (e.g. cancer, diabetes) are linked to orthorexia nervosa, while short-term concerns (e.g. fear of vomiting, choking) are connected with avoidant/restrictive food intake disorder (Donini et al., 2022). The previous preliminary evidence (Zickgraf, Ellis & Essayli, 2019) revealed that orthorexia nervosa is distinct from and has fewer features in common with avoidant-restrictive food intake disorder.

### 5.3.1 Expert Commentary: Thoughts on Orthorexia Nervosa and Avoidant/Restrictive Food Intake Disorder
by Hana Zickgraf, PhD

**Hana Zickgraf**, PhD is Research Psychologist at Rogers Behavioral Health (USA) and a licensed clinical psychologist. Her major research interests are in eating disorders, including the efficacy of exposure-based treatments, the development and refinement of assessment tools, and understanding the cognitive and physiological mechanisms responsible for the development and maintenance of eating disorders and their comorbidity with other mental health and medical conditions. She specialises in the descriptive psychopathology, assessment and treatment of avoidant/restrictive food intake disorder.

Orthorexia nervosa (ON) is a proposed diagnostic category for individuals with disordered eating characterised by a preoccupation with 'healthy' eating, rigid and self-imposed dietary rules, and distress or impairment (Donini et al., 2022). Although ON has attracted a substantial amount of research attention, it has not yet been recognised as a distinct disorder in DSM-5 or ICD-11, and its distinctness from already existing disorders is frequently called into question. Much of the research on the distinctness of ON from other diagnostic categories has focused on obsessive-compulsive disorder (e.g. Huynh et al., 2023; Zagaria et al., 2022) and other eating disorders (e.g. Atchison & Zickgraf, 2022; Zagaria et al., 2022). Meta-analytic effect sizes for the cross-sectional relationship between ON and OCD symptoms range from $r = 0.21$ to $0.40$. (Huynh et al., 2023; Zagaria et al., 2022). Zagaria and colleagues reported a meta-analytic effect size of $r = 0.36$ for ON and eating disorder (ED) symptoms. The research on the relationship between ON and EDs has focused on symptoms of anorexia nervosa, bulimia nervosa and binge eating disorder, sometimes collectively referred to as body image focused EDs. Data from one study on the cross-sectional correlation between ON and avoidant/restrictive food intake disorder (ARFID) reported effect sizes ranging from $r = 0.27$ to $0.39$ across ARFID subtypes (Zickgraf et al., 2019).

Taken together, these findings suggest that ON is related to both OCD and eating disorders but that measures of ON are not redundant with measures of OCD, ARFID or body image focused ED. Research is still needed to understand whether ON is a comorbidity or an alternate presentation or subtype of one of these diagnoses. ARFID, OCD and body image focused ED are all heterogeneous categories, inclusive of subtypes characterised by distinct symptoms and behaviours, and an argument could be made that ON falls under any of the three diagnostic umbrellas. However, if ON were to be recognised as a distinct form of psychopathology or a subtype of another disorder, it would almost certainly be classed as an eating/feeding disorder, given the centrality of maladaptive eating behaviour and/or attitudes towards food (Donini et al., 2022). Whether ON is a distinct form of disordered eating or a previously unrecognised presentation of ARFID or body image focused restrictive eating is still in question.

ARFID is characterised by restrictive disordered eating driven by aversive physiological and emotional responses to food itself or the immediate aftermath of eating (Thomas et al., 2017; Zickgraf et al., 2018). Three distinct but commonly comorbid presentations of ARFID have been described in both community and clinical samples. These involve extremely selective/neophobic ('picky') eating, leading to an inadequate dietary variety, a lack of hedonic or physiological motivation to eat, leading to undereating or skipping meals, and an intense fear of choking, vomiting, allergic reaction or another short-term consequence of eating. The diagnosis of ARFID, according to DSM-5 criteria, does not rely on the presence of a specific phenotype of restrictive eating but, rather, the absence of body image overvaluation (American Psychological Association, 2022). A patient with the proposed features of ON could meet the diagnostic criteria for ARFID if their restrictive eating caused sufficient impairment (American Psychological Association, 2022). However, ON appears to have more phenomenological similarities to the non-ARFID eating disorders.

Although they are separate diagnoses in DSM-5 and ICD-11, the body image focused EDs (and their respective spectrum diagnoses, which all fall under the category of other-specified eating disorders, OSFED) are more similar than they are different, and, under the cognitive behavioural model of eating disorders, they share a common aetiology in the overvaluation of body image, that is, shape and weight (DuBois et al., 2017; Fairburn, 2008; Wade et al., 2006). Behaviourally, all three are characterised by a cycle of restrictive eating to control body shape/weight and lapses in self-control involving breaking food rules, subjective overeating and/or objective binge eating (Fairburn, Cooper & Shafran, 2003). Because weight and shape are deeply valued, breaking restrictive rules causes shame, guilt and anxiety, which in turn negatively reinforces inappropriate compensatory behaviours like purging, fasting or excessively exercising (in bulimia nervosa and some cases of anorexia nervosa) and a redoubled commitment to restrictive eating (in all three disorders) (Fairburn, 2008; Fairburn, Cooper & Shafran, 2003). They are differentiated diagnostically by the presence/absence of clinically significant weight loss (anorexia nervosa spectrum vs. bulimia nervosa and binge eating disorder) or compensatory behaviour (bulimia nervosa or anorexia nervosa vs. binge eating disorder) (American Psychological Association, 2022).

Unlike the body image focused EDs, ARFID does not involve effortful avoidance of food that the patient finds desirable. Instead, avoided food provokes disgust and fear and/or fails to provoke hunger and enjoyment. Because avoided food is aversive or unrewarding to people with ARFID, patients do not have to use self-control to maintain their restrictive diets. This means that the effortful restricting and lapsing cycle is absent in ARFID. In contrast, a recent systematic review found that ON symptoms are correlated with both dysregulated overeating and dietary restraint, or the tendency to effortfully control one's eating by limiting intake of desirable foods (Atchison & Zickgraf, 2022). Further, ARFID is not associated with an implicit drive for thinness (Isquierdo et al., 2018), whereas several systematic reviews have found that symptoms of ON are related to a desire for weight loss, a history of dieting and, in some studies, negative body image (Atchison & Zickgraf, 2022; McComb & Mills, 2019).

Dieting, desiring weight loss and having negative feelings about one's weight and shape are all common experiences and, while associated with distress and ED risk, not inherently pathological (Bucciarini et al., 2013; Fallon et al., 2014; Latiff et al., 2018; Neumark-Sztainer et al., 2011). Similarly, ON exists on a spectrum of interest in healthy eating (Barthles et al., 2018; Donini et al., 2022). The choice to reduce intake of energy-dense foods, incorporate nutrient-rich or organic foods or increase exercise can be, and often is, adaptive both psychologically and physically. Eating a healthy diet and reaching and/or maintaining a healthy weight are very common goals, and people who undertake them usually receive approval, encouragement and support.

In contrast, the ARFID eating restrictions are not continuous with goal-directed or socially approbated behaviours. Rather, like other forms of internalising psychopathology (e.g. Strelau & Zawadzki, 2011; Ringwald et al., 2023), the physiological and behavioural characteristics of the three ARFID phenotypes are extremes of universal traits – food neophobia, the physiological regulation of food-seeking motivation, and the ability to quickly form conditioned associations from fear-provoking stimuli – expressed in ways that conflict with an individual's adaptive functioning in their environment (Thomas et al., 2017). In other words, the experience of food and eating situations as aversive in ARFID is rooted in heritable trait-like individual differences that are present early in development and not typically central to an individual's goals, values or social identity. In these regards, ARFID has more in common with OCD than it does with body image focused EDs or with ON: food avoidance is negatively reinforced by escape from aversive emotions and sensations, usually experienced as ego dystonic, and not positively reinforced by goal achievement or societal approval.

ON and the non-ARFID EDs are distinguished from nonpathological interest, drive and even obsession by the overvalued nature of the ideals involved (e.g. Vitousek & Brown, 2015). In the case of ON, these ideas and beliefs relate to health and nutrition, whereas non-ARFID EDs involve the overvaluation of weight and shape. However, the centrality of weight and shape overvaluation to disordered eating has been questioned from both modern and historical perspectives. Bhattacharya and colleagues (2022) argue that ideas about the ideal female body have shifted in recent decades, away from extreme thinness and towards lean muscularity and a 'healthy' appearance, and that ON represents a shift in the psychopathology of AN in response to this cultural change. Dell'Osso and colleagues (2016) situate modern eating disorders and ON in the medical-cultural history of psychopathology involving self-starvation, which has been documented since late antiquity but only linked to weight control motivations during the twentieth century. In the early Middle Ages in Europe, voluntary self-starvation was seen as an expression of piety, first preached by Gnostic philosophers, popularised by early Christian saints, and primarily practised by girls and women (Mavrovic, 2023). These authors make the case that rather than a drive for thinness, or even body image concern, AN and related EDs occur when acting on strongly valued beliefs or goals conflicts with eating an adequate amount or variety of food, and the change in eating behaviour is initially positively reinforced by goal attainment and validation from peers and/or society at large (Bhattacharya et al., 2022; Dell'Osso et al., 2016). Under this framework, ON, anorexia nervosa, bulimia nervosa and binge eating disorder are all manifestations of a psychopathology reflecting a derangement of value-driven and goal-oriented behaviour much older than modern beauty standards or understanding of health and nutrition. ARFID, which is neither defined by goal-directed change in eating behaviour nor overlaps with a person's values or identity, does not fit into this conceptualisation of disordered eating.

In summary, the core features that distinguish ARFID from other EDs currently conceptualised as characterised by preoccupation with body image also distinguish it from ON. The primary similarity between ARFID and ON is that distorted body image is not the driver of disordered eating. However, whereas ARFID symptoms are not related to an implicit drive for thinness, restrained eating or loss of control over eating, ON shares all of these features with body image focused EDs (e.g. Atchison & Zickgraf, 2022; McComb & Mills, 2019). When body image focused EDs are reconceptualised as disorders arising when goal achievement and following a deeply held – and maladaptively overvalued – conviction conflicts with normal eating, ON fits into this category and ARFID does not.

# Highlights

• In the early twentieth century, Donini et al. (2004) and Cartwright (2004) independently published the findings and/or observations about orthorexia nervosa for the first time. Over the last 20 years, several studies have been conducted in different countries to investigate the phenomenon of orthorexia nervosa. Nonetheless, an up-to-date overview of the clinical description of orthorexia nervosa (especially clinical diagnosis) remains challenging. To date, orthorexia nervosa as a unique diagnostic category or a mental disorder (included among the eating disorders or considered as an obsessive-compulsive disorder) lacks recognition in the DSM 5 (or DMS-5-TR) and the ICD-11. This is mainly because not enough studies have been published on the condition to distinguish it from other disorders. Despite a few existing diagnostic criteria for orthorexia nervosa (proposed by Setnick, 2013; Barthels et al., 2015a; Moroze et al., 2015; Dunn & Bratman, 2016 and Orthorexia Nervosa Task Force: Cena et al., 2019; Donini et al., 2022), none is universally accepted as a gold standard. 'Diagnostic assessment' of orthorexia nervosa is based solely on self-reported questionnaires, and individuals' biographic information and physical examination to assess physical impairment are not used in current diagnostic procedures (Strahler & Stark, 2020).

• It is a misconstruction to use the term orthorexia nervosa since the prefix 'ortho' means 'right' or 'correct' (Thorsberg, 2022). The new definition should indicate the main condition for orthorexia nervosa. Therefore, a new term called 'Salussitomania', literally meaning 'a very strong interest in health and food', has been proposed by the author of this book. To most precisely name this phenomenon, there is a need to reach a consensus on its adequate terminology. Because the term 'orthorexia nervosa' is widely used by the scientific and non-scientific communities in the present book, this term is used within the existing findings and concepts.

• The evidence has demonstrated that orthorexia nervosa reveals several similarities with anorexia nervosa and obsessive-compulsive disorder. Although orthorexia nervosa and anorexia nervosa are centred around an excessive preoccupation with food, orthorexia nervosa is distinguished from anorexia nervosa (Brytek-Matera, 2023). However, orthorexia nervosa, as it is currently operationalised and defined, aligns with anorexia nervosa more than with obsessive-compulsive disorder (Cosh et al., 2023; Zagaria et al., 2022) and with avoidant-restrictive food intake disorder (Zickgraf et al., 2019). Although some findings suggested that orthorexia nervosa could be classified on the eating disorder spectrum (Bartel et al., 2020), it is still unclear whether orthorexia nervosa represents a precursor to anorexia nervosa, an eating disorder with added health concerns or a disorder that evolves from an eating disorder (Bartel et al., 2020). The extent to which other disorders (anorexia nervosa, obsessive-compulsive disorder, avoidant-restrictive food intake disorder) are related to orthorexia nervosa will have an impact on the development of effective treatments and preventative education programmes (Huynh et al., 2023).

# Part III

# Assessment and Prevalence of Orthorexia Nervosa

# 6 Research Methods in Orthorexia Nervosa

## 6.1 First Assessment Tools for Orthorexia Nervosa

Throughout the last two decades, attempts to measure orthorexia nervosa have been ongoing. The previous systematic review (Opitz et al., 2020) provided details on 10 distinct methods for orthorexia nervosa published in multiple languages (English, German, French, Dutch or Spanish), including the Body-Image Screening Questionnaire, the Burda-Orthorexia Risk Assessment, the Bratman Orthorexia Test, the Düsseldorf Orthorexia Scale, the Eating Habits Questionnaire, the Eating Habits Questionnaire-Revised, the Orthorexia Nervosa Scale, the ORTO-15, the Scale to Measure Orthorexia in Puerto Rican Men and Women, and the Teruel Orthorexia Scale. Despite this, a gold standard does not exist for the evaluation of orthorexia nervosa (Opitz et al., 2020). Nevertheless, the ORTO-15, the Eating Habits Questionnaire and the Düsseldorf Orthorexia Scale are the first and the most frequently used self-reported questionnaires for assessing orthorexia nervosa.

### 6.1.1 The ORTO-15

The ORTO-15, developed by Donini et al. (2005), has been the most widely used tool for assessing orthorexia nervosa. It was created 'for diagnosing orthorexia nervosa' (Donini et al., 2005, p. e28). The ORTO-15 consists of 15 multiple-choice items (e.g. 'Are you willing to spend more money to have healthier food?', 'Do you feel guilty when transgressing?') scored on a 4-point Likert-type scale (from 'always' to 'never'). It is divided into three different areas: the cognitive-rational (six items), the clinical (five items) and the emotional dimensions (four items). Items that reflect an orthorexic tendency score 1 point, while those indicating normal eating behaviour score 4 points. Therefore, lower scores (below 40 points) are consistent with 'a diagnosis of orthorexia nervosa' (p. e30). At a threshold value of 40 points, the ORTO-15 reported a sensitivity value of 100%, a specificity value of 73.6%, a positive predictive value of 17.6% and a negative predictive value of 100% (Donini et al., 2004). The general sample was composed of 525 Italian participants aged over 16 years, including 404 individuals (51.8% women) for the construction of the method and 121 individuals for the validation of the ORTO-15, who completed measures of eating behaviour ('healthy' and unhealthy foods) and obsessive-phobic personality traits.

So far, the ORTO-15 has been adapted and/or validated for several languages (Table 6.1). For solving psychometric problems, several authors (see Table 6.1) have attempted to overcome limitations by shortening the ORTO-15. The modified versions of the ORTO-15, containing from 7 to 14 items, have been proposed to improve its psychometric properties. For instance, Moller

**Table 6.1** National validation studies (in English) of the ORTO-15 and its modified versions: findings from adults

| Country (in alphabetical order) | Author(s) and year | Sample (% of women) | Internal consistency of the final version of the ORTO-15: Cronbach's alpha (α) and/ or McDonald's omega (ω) | Test-retest reliability ($N_{sub\text{-}sample}$) |
|---|---|---|---|---|
| Australia | Moller, Apputhurai & Knowles, 2019 | 585 participants (82.4%) | $\alpha_{7\text{-item version}} = 0.83$ | N/A |
| Brazil | Alvarenga et al., 2012 | 392 dietitians (93%) | $\alpha_{12\text{-item version}} = 0.39$ | N/A |
| China | Li et al., 2022 | 1,289 university students (37.9%) | $\alpha_{15\text{-item version}} = 0.79$ | ICC with an interval of 2 weeks= 0.79 ($N$= 38) |
| France | Babeau et al., 2020 | 768 adults (84.77%) | $\alpha_{12\text{-item version}} = 0.73$ | N/A |
| Germany | Missbach et al., 2015 | 1,029 adults (74.6%) | $\alpha_{9\text{-item version}} = 0.67$ | N/A |
| Greece | Gonidakis et al., 2021 | 120 university students (N/A) | $\alpha_{15\text{-item version}} = 0.7$ | ICC with an interval of 2 weeks= 0.75 ($N$= 20) |
| Greece | Gkiouras et al., 2022 | 848 adults (65.68%) | $\omega_{15\text{-item version}} = 0.70$ | N/A |
| Hungary | Varga et al., 2014 | 810 university students (89.4%) | $\alpha_{11\text{-item version}} = 0.82$ | N/A |
| Lebanon | Haddad et al., 2020 | 806 adults (77.3%) | $\alpha_{15\text{-item version}} = 0.82$ | N/A |

## Table 6.1 (cont.)

| Country (in alphabetical order) | Author(s) and year | Sample (% of women) | Internal consistency of the final version of the ORTO-15: Cronbach's alpha (α) and/ or McDonald's omega (ω) | Test-retest reliability ($N_{sub\text{-}sample}$) |
|---|---|---|---|---|
| Mexico | Tena et al., 2021 | 911 university students (65.4%) | $α_{14\text{-item version}} = 0.78$ | N/A |
| Poland | Brytek-Matera et al., 2014 | 400 university students and administrative and teaching personnel (85.25%) | $α_{9\text{-item version}} = 0.64$ | N/A |
| Spain | Roncero, Barrada & Perpiñá, 2017 | 242 university students (63.2%) | $α_{11\text{-item version}} = 0.74$ | $r = 0.92$ |
| Spain | Parra-Fernández et al., 2018b | 454 university students (64.98%) | $α_{11\text{-item version}} = 0.80$ | N/A |

Note: ICC: intra-class correlation.

and colleagues (2019) conducted confirmatory factor analyses of the 15-, 11- and 9-item versions of the ORTO-15. They concluded that none of the three versions showed acceptable model fit (Goodness of Fit Index (GFI) > 0.90, Comparative Fit Index (CFI) > 0.90, Tucker-Lewis Index (TLI) > 0.90 and Root Mean Square Error of Approximation (RMSEA) < 0.08). With removing two items from the 9-item version, the ORTO-7 was proposed (Moller et al., 2019).

A previous critical literature review with a systematic search (Valente, Syurina & Donini, 2019) set out some of the most common criticisms of the ORTO-15: weak psychometric properties (the validity and reliability; e.g. Alvarenga et al., 2012; McComb & Mills, 2019; Niedzielski & Kaźmierczak-Wojtaś, 2021; Roncero, Barrada & Perpiñá, 2017) and overestimation of the prevalence of orthorexia nervosa (e.g. Dunn & Bratman, 2016; Cena et al., 2019; Reynolds, 2018). The previous and recent studies advised against using the ORTO-15 (e.g. Gkiouras et al., 2022; Opitz et al., 2020; Meule et al., 2020; Missbach et al., 2017). Although the shortened versions of the ORTO-15 report various acceptable psychometric properties using the group with which it was developed, their multiplicity of the modified versions of the ORTO-15 can lead to the inability to compare the research findings. Furthermore, it has been suggested that the ORTO-15 detects healthy eating (Dunn et al., 2016), normative healthy eating behaviour and normative health-conscious (Heiss et al., 2019) and not whether the behaviour is pathological (Dunn et al., 2016), thus it is not an adequate scale to detect orthorexic behaviours and attitudes (Mitrofanova et al., 2021). Therefore, to assess orthorexia nervosa, the abandonment of the ORTO-15 (Zickgraf, 2020) and the use of other measures is recommended.

### 6.1.2 The Eating Habits Questionnaire

The Eating Habits Questionnaire (EHQ), developed by Gleaves, Graham and Ambwani (2013), '*assesses the cognitions, behaviours, and feelings related to an extreme focus on healthy eating*' (p. 1). The EHQ consists of 21 multiple-choice items scored on a 4-point Likert-type scale (from 'false, not at all true' to 'very true'). The EHQ is composed of three different factors: knowledge of healthy eating (5 items; e.g. 'I am more informed than others about healthy eating'), problems associated with healthy eating (12 items; e.g. 'I am distracted by thoughts of eating healthily') and feeling positively about healthy eating (4 items; e.g. 'Eating the way I do gives me a sense of satisfaction'). Higher scores are indicative of knowledge of healthy eating, problems associated with healthy eating and orthorexia, as well as positive feelings associated with healthy eating. Each of the subscales of the EHQ displays good internal consistency ($\alpha_{Knowledge} = 0.82$, $\alpha_{Problems} = 0.90$ and $\alpha_{Feelings} = 0.86$) and acceptable test-retest reliability ($r_{Knowledg} = 0.81$, $r_{Problems} = 0.81$ and $r_{Feelings} = 0.72$). The general sample was composed of 387 US undergraduate students, including 174 individuals (aged 18–38 years; 68% women) for the factor structure of the method and 213 individuals (aged 18–48 years; 65% women) for the validation of the method. Problems associated with healthy eating were linked with eating disorder pathology, obsessive-compulsive symptoms, negative affect and depressed mood rather than with personality functioning, social desirability or general psychopathology. Knowledge of healthy eating and feeling positively about healthy eating was related to conscientiousness and unrelated to general psychopathology, depression and self-deceptive enhancement. A high statistical overlap was found between the EHQ, a measure of problematic preoccupations with healthy eating and the Eating Attitudes Test-26, which is a measure of eating disorder pathology. '*This may mean that the EHQ is measuring the same construct as the EAT-26, but more poorly regarding its predictive power, or alternatively may mean that "ON"* [orthorexia nervosa] *is simply a sub-facet of AN* [anorexia nervosa]' (Gleaves, Graham & Ambwani, 2013, p. 13). Similar to anorexia nervosa, orthorexia nervosa may be a multidimensional construct. However, not all dimensions of orthorexia nervosa may be harmful (Gleaves, Graham & Ambwani, 2013).

So far, the EHQ has been adopted and/or validated in two English-speaking and five non-English-speaking countries (Table 6.2).

Table 6.2 National validation studies (in English) of the EHQ: findings from adults

| Country (in alphabetical order) | Author(s) and year | Sample (% of women) | Internal consistency: Cronbach's alpha ($\alpha$) and/or McDonald's omega ($\omega$) | Test-retest reliability ($N_{sub-sample}$) |
|---|---|---|---|---|
| Australia | Mohamed Halim et al., 2020 | 286 female adults (100%) | $\alpha_{Total} = 0.89$<br>$\alpha_{Diet\ superiority} = 0.80$<br>$\alpha_{Dietary\ restriction} = 0.72$<br>$\alpha_{Healthy\ eating\ cognitions} = 0.77$<br>$\alpha_{Social\ impairment} = 0.77$ | N/A |
| France | Godefroy, Trinchera & Dorard, 2021 | 1,887 adults (89.67%) | $\alpha_{Total} = 0.89$<br>$\alpha_{Positive\ feeling\ of\ control} = 0.76$<br>$\alpha_{Problems\ of\ attention\ control\ and\ social\ relationships} = 0.75$<br>$\alpha_{Rigid\ eating\ behaviour} = 0.82$ | N/A |
| Greece | Bali et al., 2023 | 551 adults from the general population (92.2%) | $\alpha_{Total} = N/A$<br>$\alpha_{Feelings} = 0.82$<br>$\alpha_{Knowledge} = 0.80$<br>$\alpha_{Problems} = 0.82$ | No statistically significant difference between the measurements of the first and the post 2 weeks |
| Lebanon | Hallit et al., 2021 | 456 adults (56.2%) | $\alpha_{Orthorexia\ nervosa} = 0.89$<br>$\alpha_{Healthy\ orthorexia} = 0.86$ | N/A |

Table 6.2 (cont.)

| Country (in alphabetical order) | Author(s) and year | Sample (% of women) | Internal consistency: Cronbach's alpha (α) and/or McDonald's omega (ω) | Test-retest reliability ($N_{sub-sample}$) |
|---|---|---|---|---|
| Poland | Brytek-Matera, Plasonja & Décamps, 2020 | 967 individuals from the general population (77.2%) | $\alpha_{Total} = 0.88$<br>$\alpha_{Feelings\ and\ Behaviours} = 0.81$<br>$\alpha_{Knowledge} = 0.85$<br>$\alpha_{Problems} = 0.81$ | N/A |
| Spain | Parra-Fernández et al., 2021 | 487 university students (Sample 1 = 81.9%; Sample 2 = 52.2%) | $\alpha_{Total} = 0.90$<br>$\alpha_{Feelings} = 0.77$<br>$\alpha_{Knowledge} = 0.78$<br>$\alpha_{Problems} = 0.85$<br>$\omega_{Total} = 0.93$<br>$\omega_{Feelings} = 0.77$<br>$\omega_{Knowledge} = 0.82$<br>$\omega_{Problems} = 0.87$ | N/A |
| United States | Oberle, Samaghabadi & Hughes, 2017 | 459 college students (80.8%) | $\alpha_{Total} = 0.90$<br>$\alpha_{Feelings} = 0.73$<br>$\alpha_{Behaviours} = 0.87$<br>$\alpha_{Problems} = 0.79$ | N/A |

The EHQ is a promising alternative to the ORTO-15 for assessing orthorexia nervosa (Oberle, Samaghabadi & Hughes, 2017). Only one criticism was raised about the tool (Valente, Syurina & Donini, 2019), namely the lack of criterion validity (that is, an estimate of the extent to which a tool agrees with another tool measuring the same phenomenon) (Oberle, Samaghabadi & Hughes, 2017).

### 6.1.3 The Düsseldorf Orthorexia Scale

The Düsseldorf Orthorexia Scale (DOS), developed by Barthels, Meyer and Pietrowsky (2015b), assesses 'orthorexic eating behaviour' (p. 97). The DOS consists of 10 multiple-choice items (e.g. 'I can only enjoy eating foods considered healthy', 'I feel upset after eating unhealthy foods') scored on a 4-point Likert-type scale (from 'this applies to me' to 'this does not apply to me'). The maximum score is 40 points. The cut-off score of 30 is used to identify orthorexic eating behaviour, while a score between 25 and 29 indicates a risk of orthorexia nervosa. The DOS demonstrates good internal consistency ($\alpha = 84$) and acceptable test-retest reliability ($r = 0.79$). The general sample comprised 1,340 German students and employed people over 18 years (70% women). Orthorexic eating behaviour, measured by the DOS, was associated with psychological and behavioural symptoms of eating disorders (namely drive for thinness, bulimia and body dissatisfaction), health anxiety and hypochondriacal worries as well as with the subjective importance of healthy eating and self-rated health of eating behaviour.

So far, the DOS has been adopted and/or validated in one English-speaking country and eight non-English-speaking countries (Table 6.3).

Table 6.3 National validation studies (in English) of the DOS: findings from adults

| Country (in alphabetical order) | Author(s) and year | Sample (% of women) | Internal consistency: Cronbach's alpha ($\alpha$) and/ or McDonald's omega ($\omega$) | Test-retest reliability ($N_{sub\text{-}sample}$) |
|---|---|---|---|---|
| Brazil | Souza et al., 2021 | 486 dietitians and nutrition college students (91.6%) | $\alpha = 0.79$ | ICC* $= 0.77$ ($N = 159$) |
| China | He et al., 2019 | 1,075 under-graduate students (52.7%) | $\alpha = 0.84$ | ICC with an interval of 4 weeks $= 0.77$ ($N = 101$) |
| France | Lasson, Barthels & Raynal, 2021 | 3,235 university students (89.67%) | $\omega = 0.87$ | N/A |
| Italy | Cerolini et al., 2022 | 422 university students (71.8%) | $\alpha = 0.88$ | N/A |
| Italy | Aloi et al., 2023 | 521 individuals from the general population (62.6%) | $\omega = 0.87$ | N/A |
| Lebanon | Hallit et al., 2021 | 456 adults (56.2%) | $\alpha = 0.87$ | N/A |

Table 6.3 (cont.)

| Country (in alphabetical order) | Author(s) and year | Sample (% of women) | Internal consistency: Cronbach's alpha (α) and/or McDonald's omega (ω) | Test-retest reliability $(N_{sub-sample})$ |
|---|---|---|---|---|
| Poland | Brytek-Matera, 2021b | 412 university students (77.2%) | α = 0.84 ω = 0.84 | N/A |
| Portugal | Ferreira & Coimbra, 2021 | 513 individuals from the general population (88.5%) | α = 0.86 | N/A |
| Spain | Parra-Fernández et al., 2019a | 492 university students (N/A) | α = 0.84 | N/A |
| United States | Chard et al., 2019 | 384 under-graduate students (69.5%) | α = 0.88 | N/A |

Note: ICC: intra-class correlation; * Time interval is not presented.

Like the EHQ, the DOS is an internally reliable self-report measure. Both questionnaires are characterised by unidimensionality, good internal reliability and satisfactory construct validity (Meule et al., 2020). The general criticism of the DOS has been an issue relating to the fact that this measure does not seem to be able to distinguish between anorexia nervosa and orthorexia nervosa (Barthels et al., 2017). Moreover, the previous systematic review and reliability generalisation (Opitz et al., 2020) found that the dimensionality of the DOS remains inconclusive, with one factor indicating poor fit.

## 6.2 Novel Assessment Tools for Orthorexia Nervosa

Three novel measures, namely the Teruel Orthorexia Scale (Barrada & Roncero, 2018), the Barcelona Orthorexia Nervosa Scale (Bauer et al., 2019) and the Orthorexia Nervosa Inventory (Oberle, De Nadai & Madrid, 2021) were developed in the last five years (after the publication of the diagnostic criteria by Dunn and Bratman, 2016).

### 6.2.1 The Teruel Orthorexia Scale

The Teruel Orthorexia Scale (TOS), developed by Barrada & Roncero (2018), assesses 'two related, although differentiable, aspects of orthorexia' (p. 289): orthorexia nervosa (8 items; e.g. 'Thoughts about healthy eating do not let me concentrate on other tasks') and healthy orthorexia (9 items; e.g. 'I feel good when I eat healthy food'). *'Healthy orthorexia evaluates the tendency to eat healthy food and interest in doing so. It represents a healthy interest with diet, which is independent of psychopathology (eating disorders, obsessive-compulsive disorder and negative affect), and even inversely associated with it. People with high scores on this factor are interested in a healthy diet, they spend a considerable amount of time and money buying, planning and preparing healthy food. This interest is in accordance with their self, as they describe their attitudes almost as a way of life. This factor represents the so-called orthorexia (non-nervosa). On the other hand, orthorexia nervosa assesses the negative social and emotional impact of trying to achieve a rigid way of eating. This dimension represents a pathological preoccupation with a healthy diet, which corresponds with the so-called orthorexia nervosa. People scoring high on this factor are highly concerned with and overwhelmed by their preoccupations, which lead them to negative consequences such as self-punishment, social isolation and guilt. This factor is associated with obsessive-compulsive symptoms, but mainly with eating symptoms (…)'* (Barrada & Roncero, 2018, p. 289). The TOS consists of 17 multiple-choice items scored on a 4-point Likert-type scale (from 'completely disagree' to 'completely agree'). Higher scores are indicative of orthorexic symptoms. The TOS indicates good internal consistency ($\alpha_{\text{Orthorexia Nervosa}}$ = 0.81 and $\alpha_{\text{Healthy Orthorexia}}$ = 0.85) and acceptable test-retest reliability ($r_{\text{Orthorexia Nervosa}}$ =0.82 and $r_{\text{Healthy Orthorexia}}$= 0.73). The general sample comprised 942 mainly Spanish university students (aged 18–66 years; 76% women; 148 provided responses in a retest 18 months later). Orthorexia nervosa was positively related to symptoms and concerns characteristic of eating disorders (the highest association with dieting and bulimia), concern over mistakes, obsessive-compulsive symptoms, negative affect and negatively related to positive appraisals of one's physical appearance. These associations were not altered when controlling for healthy orthorexia. Barrada and Roncero (2018) identified some limitations: the sample being drawn from a population of students, the predominance of women (which limits the representability of the results) and the use of the self-reported questionnaires. It has also been indicated that the cross-cultural validity of the TOS remains uncertain (Chace & Kluck, 2022), and there is a lack of cut-off points for this measure (Roberto da Silva et al., 2021).

So far, the TOS has been adapted and/or validated in five countries (Table 6.4).

Table 6.4 National validation studies (in English) of the TOS: findings from adults

| Country (in alphabetical order) | Author(s) and year | Sample (% of women) | Internal consistency: Cronbach's alpha (α) and/or McDonald's omega (ω) and/or the composite reliability indicator (ρc) and/or the nonlinear structural equation modelling reliability (ρNL) coefficients | Test-retest reliability ($N_{\text{sub-sample}}$) |
|---|---|---|---|---|
| Brazil | Roberto da Silva et al., 2021 | 226 gym users (36.3%) | $\rho NL_{\text{Orthorexia Nervosa}} = 0.82$; $\rho NL_{\text{Healthy Orthorexia}} = 0.83$<br>$\alpha_{\text{Orthorexia Nervosa}} = 0.91$; $\alpha_{\text{Healthy Nervosa}} = 0.90$<br>$\omega_{\text{Orthorexia Nervosa}} = 0.87$; $\omega_{\text{Healthy Orthorexia}} = 0.78$ | N/A |
| Canada | Maïano et al., 2022 | 296 adults (85.1%) | $\omega_{\text{Orthorexia Nervosa}} = 0.87$; $\omega_{\text{Healthy Orthorexia}} = 0.92$ | N/A |
| France | Lasson et al., 2023 | 799 adults (82.9%) | $\alpha_{\text{Orthorexia Nervosa}} = 0.81$; $\alpha_{\text{Healthy Orthorexia}} = 0.83$ | N/A |
| Italy | Falgares et al., 2023 | 782 adults (82%) | $\rho c_{\text{Orthorexia Nervosa}} = 0.91$; $\rho c_{\text{Healthy Orthorexia}} = 0.90$ | ICC with an interval of 2 weeks $_{\text{Orthorexia Nervosa}} = 0.83$<br>ICC with an interval of 2 weeks $_{\text{Healthy Orthorexia}} = 0.84$ ($N = 144$) |
| United States | Chace & Kluck, 2022 | 304 undergraduate students (71.7%) | $\alpha_{\text{Orthorexia Nervosa}} = 0.86$; $\alpha_{\text{Healthy Orthorexia}} = 0.88$ | N/A |

Notably, the lack of consensus about the definition of pathological healthy eating versus healthy eating involves contradictions (Opitz et al., 2020). On the one hand, feelings of superiority regarding one's healthy diet are recognised and considered as a core feature of orthorexia nervosa (Bratman & Knight, 2000). On the other hand, they are classified as part of 'healthy orthorexia' in the TOS (Barrada & Roncero, 2018). In the author's opinion, we are not confronted with the problem in terms of the understanding that the presence of distress and clinical impairment and their impact on daily functioning indicate abnormal conditions, thus related to engagement with healthy eating with a pathological approach to healthy eating. The issue of unequivocal definition and the objective way we could measure two distinct dimensions (healthy eating and pathological preoccupation with healthy eating) remains a problem. Thus, the current contradictions in the conceptualisation of orthorexia nervosa (Opitz et al., 2020) and the lack of one universally accepted definition of pathological healthy eating may mean that we are not describing and/or investigating the same construct.

### 6.2.2 The Barcelona Orthorexia Scale

The Barcelona Orthorexia Scale (BOS), developed by Bauer and colleagues (2019), assesses 'psychological characteristics' of orthorexia nervosa (p. 249). The BOS was based on a Delphi study methodology (a three-round) including international experts (researchers and/or clinicians) on eating disorders ($N = 292$) and orthorexia nervosa ($N = 52$). The diagnostic criteria by Dunn and Bratman (2016) and the scientific literature (Brytek-Matera, 2012; Barthels, Meyer & Pietrowsky, 2015; Moroze et al., 2015) provided the basis on which the items were developed (Bauer et al., 2019). The BOS consists of 64 items (e.g. 'I try to never break any of my own dietary rules', 'I feel rejected or under-valued by my social environment due to my eating habits'). It is composed of six content areas measuring psychological aspects of orthorexia nervosa: cognitive domain (14 items), emotional domain (16 items), behavioural domain (14 items), negative consequences – health (6 items), negative consequences – impairment in social or academic functioning (9 items) and differential diagnosis domain – orthorexia versus other eating disorders (5 items). Bauer and colleagues (2019) identified some limitations. First, the Spanish expert panel had significantly less knowledge about orthorexia nervosa than the English ones. Second, not all participants were experts in orthorexia nervosa. However, some of them were experts in eating disorders and were working in the clinical setting. For these reasons, most of the experts (57%) did not have published papers on orthorexia nervosa. Third, the experts were all authors and co-authors of the studies found in the literature research. Therefore, it is possible that students and/or statistical consultants could have included and introduced bias in validating the items. Nevertheless, the BOS, based on the diagnostic criteria for orthorexia nervosa (Dunn & Bratman, 2016), and through expert consensus, has demonstrated adequate content validity (Bauer et al., 2019). So far, the BOS has been solely adapted and validated to the Spanish language used in Spain (Navarro et al., 2023). The sample was composed of 550 individuals from the general population (aged 18–70 years; 81.1% women) who completed measures of symptoms and concerns characteristic of eating disorders as well as eating behaviours, namely emotional intake, external intake and restrictive behaviour. The initial BOS demonstrated excellent internal consistency ($\alpha$ = 0.949) and good test-retest reliability ($r$ = 0.876). The final version of the BOS was composed of 35 items, including five factors: behavioural area ($\alpha$ = 0.851), preoccupation about healthy food ($\alpha$ = 0.902), attitudes and beliefs about food ($\alpha$ = 0.804), vital achievement ($\alpha$ = 0.836) and emotional distress ($\alpha$ = 0.935). It also had an excellent internal consistency ($\alpha$ = 0.953) and good test-retest reliability ($r$ = 0.877). Therefore, the BOS, as a valid and reliable measure, could be useful for assessing the psychological characteristics of orthorexia nervosa in the general population.

## 6.2.3 The Orthorexia Nervosa Inventory

The Orthorexia Nervosa Inventory (ONI), developed by Oberle, De Nadai and Madrid (2021) assesses symptomatology of orthorexia nervosa 'that includes an adequate number of items to assess each of the four consensus diagnostic criteria for orthorexia nervosa' (Oberle, De Nadai & Madrid, 2021, p. 611), including behaviours and preoccupation with 'healthy' eating (criterion A), emotional distress resulting from violations of their dietary rules (criterion B), physical impairments resulting from nutritional deficiencies (criterion C) and psychosocial impairments resulting from the other criteria (criterion D). The ONI consists of 24 multiple-choice items scored on a 4-point Likert-type scale (from 'not at all true' to 'very true'). In the case of criteria A, B and C, a few items modified from the EHQ and/ or the DOS were included. In contrast, all novel items were presented in the case of criterion C. The ONI is composed of three different factors: behaviours (9 items, e.g. 'I follow a healthy diet with many rules'), impairments (10 items; e.g. 'My cleanses or fasts have become more frequent or severe over time') and emotions (5 items; e.g. 'I feel much guilt or self-loathing when I stray from my healthy diet'). Higher scores indicate greater orthorexic symptomatology. The ONI demonstrates excellent internal consistency ($\alpha_{Total}$ = 0.94, $\alpha_{Behaviours}$ = 0.89, $\alpha_{Impairments}$ = 0.90, $\alpha_{Emotions}$ = 0.88) and excellent 2-week test-retest reliability ($r_{Total}$ = 0.91, $r_{Behaviours}$ = 0.87, $r_{Impairments}$ = 0.86, $r_{Emotions}$ = 0.87). The general sample comprised 847 US adults (aged 18–75 years; 82% women). The ONI and each of its scales exhibited positive associations with health-related behaviours, namely aerobic exercise, the compulsive need to structure exercise activities and the compulsive need to exercise. Additionally, the ONI was positively linked to healthy eating behaviours regarding the consumption of vegetables and fruits and negatively associated with the consumption of meat, dairy products, sweetened beverages and sweets. Moreover, the ONI and each of its scales were also significantly positively associated with symptoms and concerns characteristic of eating disorders and obsessive-compulsive symptoms, as well as depression-related problems. Regarding limitations, the selection of items specifically linked to the consensus diagnostic criteria for orthorexia nervosa is prone to biases due to the subjective choice of the items, which impacts the interpretability of the final scale. Another limitation relates to the inclusion of participants with a self-reported diagnosis of an eating disorder in the construction of a new measure. Finally, regarding the recommended 'diagnostic' criterion, the proposed cut-off score for the ONI (a mean Likert rating of 3 'mainly true' equates to a minimum total score of 72) cannot be an indication of a diagnosis of orthorexia nervosa. Rather, this value should only be used to assess the risk of orthorexia nervosa individually and/or to examine similarities and differences between different populations (Oberle, De Nadai & Madrid, 2021).

So far, the ONI has been adapted and/or validated in two non-English-speaking countries (Table 6.5).

Table 6.5 National validation studies (in English) of the ONI: findings from adults

| Country (in alphabetical order) | Author(s) and year | Sample (% of women) | Internal consistency: Cronbach's alpha ($\alpha$) and/or McDonald's omega ($\omega$) | Test-retest reliability ($N_{\text{sub-sample}}$) |
|---|---|---|---|---|
| Italy | Zagaria et al., 2023 | 879 adults (56.9%) | $\omega_{\text{Behaviours}} = 0.88$ $\omega_{\text{Impairments}} = 0.88$ $\omega_{\text{Emotions}} = 0.91$ | N/A |
| Turkey | Kaya, Uzdil & Çakıroğlu, 2022 | 710 adults (70.8%) | $\alpha_{\text{Total}} = 0.90$ $\alpha_{\text{Behaviours}} = 0.82$ $\alpha_{\text{Impairments}} = 0.84$ $\alpha_{\text{Emotions}} = 0.80$ | N/A |

Currently, the ONI is the only measure including items about physical impairments (one of the consensus diagnostic criteria for orthorexia nervosa) and other diagnostic criteria (A, B and D) that researchers have agreed upon. Combining various expert opinions in the construction approaches of the ONI (Opitz et al., 2020) may yield satisfactory results and improve the research surrounding orthorexia nervosa.

## 6.3 Revision of the Existing Assessment Tool: The ORTO-R

The ORTO-R, a new revised version of the ORTO-15, was proposed by Rogoza and Donini (2021) to assess orthorexic thoughts and behaviours dimensionally, omitting the categorical diagnosis. The ORTO-R consists of six multiple-choice items (e.g. 'Would you agree that eating healthy food increases your self-esteem?', 'In the last three months, did the thoughts of food make you feel guilt, ashamed and anxious?') scored on a 5-point Likert-type scale (from 'never' to 'always'). Reverse scoring was changed, with higher scores indicating higher orthorexic thoughts and behaviours. Furthermore, the order of items was randomly changed to reduce the potential effects of the method bias. Taking account of the specific limitations of the ORTO-15 (e.g. the impossibility of conducting tests of measurement invariance due to the unstable factorial structure of the ORTO-15, the counterintuitive ways to score, where low scores indicate higher pathology), the authors (Rogoza & Donini, 2021) used the original dataset for the development of ORTO-15 (Donini et al., 2005) to assess its factorial structure and propose its revision, the ORTO-R. The reliability of the ORTO-R was found to be acceptable ($\omega = 0.75$). A few limitations were considered when interpreting the ORTO-R (Rogoza & Donini, 2021). The items of the ORTO-R pertain to all diagnostic criteria of orthorexia nervosa (A, B and D), except physical impairments related to nutritional deficiencies (criterion C). Even though the two-factor model represented almost an exact fit to the model with the method factor, the authors opted to apply a unidimensional model. Finally, the estimates of internal consistency were not very convincing. The small number of items might result in underestimating obtained internal consistencies in future studies. Therefore the authors endorse using the coefficient omega (Rogoza & Donini, 2021).

So far, the ORTO-R has been adapted and/or validated in five non-English-speaking countries (Table 6.6).

The ORTO-R overcomes the main limitations of the ORTO-15 (Rogoza & Donini, 2021) and outperforms the TOS with regard to the strength of the correlation with (rigid, self-critical and narcissistic) perfectionism and depression

**Table 6.6** National validation studies (in English) of the ORTO-R: findings from adults

| Country (in alphabetical order) | Author(s) and year | Sample (% of women) | Internal consistency: Cronbach's alpha (α) and/ or McDonald's omega (ω) | Test-retest reliability ($N_{sub-sample}$) |
|---|---|---|---|---|
| China | Li et al., 2022 | 1,084 university students (68.1%) | α = 0.77 | ICC with an interval of 2 weeks = 0.82 (N= 48) |
| Greece | Gkiouras et al., 2022 | 848 adults (65.68%) | ω = 0.65 | N/A |
| Lebanon | Rogoza et al., 2022 | 363 university students (61.7%) | α =0.78 | N/A |
| Poland | Brytek-Matera et al., 2023 | 478 university students (87.9%) (study 2) | α = 0.71 (study 2) | N/A |
| | | 1, 529 adults (51.9% women) (study 3) | α = 0.82 (study 3) | |
| Turkey | Özdengül et al., 2021 | 877 recreational and competitive athletes and sedentary individuals (N/A) | ω = 0.72 | N/A |

Note: ICC: intra-class correlation.

symptoms (Rogoza et al., 2022). Notably, the ORTO-R is not intended to assess the prevalence of orthorexia nervosa but to evaluate orthorexic behaviours (Rogoza & Donini, 2021).

## 6.4 Screening Questions for Orthorexia Nervosa

### 6.4.1 The Orthorexia Self-Test

The first screening instrument for orthorexia nervosa was developed by Bratman and Knight (2000). The Orthorexia Self-Test, a 'yes' or 'no' 'ten-question quiz' (p. 57) (e.g. 'Do you keep getting stricter with yourself?', 'Does your diet socially isolate you?') was created as a personal risk assessment, not as an assessment tool for orthorexia nervosa (Dunn & Bratman, 2016). Therefore, it

**Table 6.7** Orthorexia nervosa screening questions

1. Do you think that eating you consider healthy has a dominant position in your life?
2. Do you constantly think about being healthy?
3. Does non-compliance with the food rules you consider healthy affect how you feel about yourself?
4. Do the food rules you consider healthy affect your interpersonal relationships or other areas of your life?
5. Is the purity of the food you consume more important than its quantity?
6. Do you ever experience feelings of guilt, shame, anxiety and/or distress due to the dietary rules you consider healthy?
7. Have you ever experienced how food rules you consider healthy impact your mental and physical well-being?

Note: A 'yes' (1 point) to each question is classified as an abnormal response.

lacks basic psychometric properties. Despite this, it has been used in several studies (see Valente, Syurina & Donini, 2019; Opitz et al., 2020).

### 6.4.2 Orthorexia Nervosa Screening Questions

There is a need for a screening tool to assess 'orthorexia nervosa risk' to determine whether an individual is experiencing symptoms of this condition and whether further testing is warranted or not to make an orthorexia nervosa diagnosis. To measure orthorexia nervosa symptomatology, Orthorexia Nervosa Screening Questions might be potentially useful (Table 6.7). These seven questions addressing the main features of orthorexia nervosa are aligned with the existing diagnostic criteria of orthorexia nervosa (Dunn & Bratman, 2016).

A score of 6 or greater is likely to indicate a risk of orthorexia nervosa.

These questions have been used in the therapeutic practice of the author of this book with individuals having disordered eating behaviours to detect the risk of orthorexia nervosa. However, it is noteworthy that they have to be (pilot) tested and validated empirically.

## 6.5 Expert Commentary: Thoughts on Orthorexia Nervosa and Its Assessment

by Adrian Meule, PhD

**Adrian Meule**, PhD is a researcher at the University of Regensburg, Germany. His major research interests are eating behaviour, eating disorders and obesity, about which he has published more than 100 scientific articles. He is the founder of the specialty section *Eating Behavior* of the journal *Frontiers in Psychology*, served as section editor for *Food Addiction* of the journal *Current Addiction Reports* and is currently on the editorial boards of *Mental Health Science* and *Obesity Science and Practice*. He has authored the book *Diagnostik von Essverhalten* [in German; engl. *Assessment of Eating Behavior*] and is editor of the book *Assessment of Eating Behavior*.

Affiliation: Department of Psychology, University of Regensburg, Regensburg, Germany.

Establishing validity of new concepts in the area of behavioural and mental disorders is not an easy task. Usually, a first step is to develop a questionnaire for measuring that concept. But how can validity of that questionnaire be shown when there is no other instrument that has already been established for assessing this novel concept? This is an inherent problem when new disorders are proposed that often results in biased interpretation of research findings. For example, a researcher may correlate the questionnaire with existing questionnaires that measure other but related concepts. Yet, the interpretation of whether the resulting correlations indicate validity of the new concept (and the questionnaire) is largely driven by one's a priori views. This process has been observed across different fields of study, for example when examining research on behavioural addictions such as excessive sexual activity, buying, gambling, working or exercising (Billieux et al., 2015). In relation to food and eating, similar debates have surrounded the concept of 'food addiction' (Lacroix, Tavares & von Ranson, 2017; Vainik & Meule, 2017) and other syndromes (Vandereycken, 2011).

Research on orthorexia was started off just like this. In their book *Health Food Junkies*, Bratman and Knight (2000) included a list of possible symptoms for which readers could answer for themselves whether they applied to them and, if so, may indicate the presence of so-called orthorexia nervosa. However, this was actually not a questionnaire intended for use in scientific studies, although some researchers later used it as such. The first questionnaire that was intentionally developed for scientific purposes was the ORTO-15 by Donini and colleagues (2005). Yet, nearly two decades of research have clearly shown that this questionnaire is not psychometrically sound and, thus, not suitable for the measurement of orthorexic eating tendencies (Meule et al., 2020; Missbach, Dunn & König, 2017).

To date, several other questionnaires have been developed: the Eating Habits Questionnaire (Gleaves, Graham & Ambwani, 2013), the Düsseldorf Orthorexia Scale (DOS; Barthels, Meyer & Pietrowsky, 2015), the Barcelona Orthorexia Scale (Bauer et al., 2019), the Teruel Orthorexia Scale (Barrada & Roncero, 2018) and the Orthorexia Nervosa Inventory (ONI; Oberle, De Nadai

& Madrid, 2021). Of these, the DOS has been the most widely used in recent years and appears to have much more favourable psychometric properties than the ORTO-15 (Oberle & Noebel, 2023). Yet, a crucial feature of all behavioural and mental disorders is that their symptoms are accompanied by a clinically significant impairment or distress, an aspect that is only mildly covered in the DOS. The ONI, for example, puts a stronger emphasis on this by including several items for assessing physical and psychosocial impairments that result from orthorexic behaviours.

When using these questionnaires, however, it has been noted that what they measure may not be sufficiently distinct from other conditions. When using the DOS, for example, large overlaps have been found with established eating disorder diagnoses and the scale positively correlates with weight and shape concerns although conceptualisations of orthorexia nervosa posit that orthorexic eating is not driven by such concerns (Meule & Voderholzer, 2021; Strahler et al., 2018; Strahler & Stark, 2018). Thus, even when accepting that existing questionnaires validly assess orthorexic eating, it appears that indications for discriminant validity – that is, that they measure a construct that can be clearly differentiated from existing constructs – are meagre. Therefore, while newer measures such as the DOS or the ONI surely can be used for the investigation of orthorexic eating tendencies, they cannot really answer the question of whether orthorexia nervosa is an own diagnostic entity that is distinct from established eating disorder diagnoses such as anorexia nervosa. A crucial next step in research on orthorexia will be the development of a standardised interview that experts in the field have agreed upon. When such an interview has been developed that yields a clear diagnosis of orthorexia nervosa while at the same time excludes the presence of other eating disorders such as anorexia nervosa, then such an interview could be used for validating the questionnaire measures mentioned above.

As is described in this book, there are, of course, humans who display an eating behaviour that is marked by an excessive focus on healthy eating that goes awry. Such orthorexic tendencies can be measured with one of the newer questionnaires such as the DOS or the ONI. However, these questionnaires fall short when it comes to proving whether orthorexia nervosa can actually be considered an own diagnostic entity that is distinct from established eating disorder diagnoses. If someone shows an excessive focus on healthy eating, that is, has high scores on the said questionnaires, an important next question is whether this is a clinically relevant condition that requires treatment and, next, whether this condition is different (and, thus, whether its treatment should be different) from other conditions that are included in current diagnostic manuals and for which specific treatments exist. Unfortunately, this is a much more complex issue that cannot be solved by the administration of questionnaire measures alone.

# 7    Prevalence of Orthorexia Nervosa

For more than two decades since the description of orthorexia nervosa, its prevalence has been investigated in various subgroups and populations worldwide using different measurement tools and the value of cut-off points (See Chapter 6). Due to the limitations regarding the lack of reliable and valid assessment tools as well as the absence of detailed diagnostic criteria, the assessment of the prevalence of orthorexia nervosa presents a difficult challenge. The prevalence of orthorexia nervosa depends on the study group, country and the instrument being used. In the previous literature review (Niedzielski & Kaźmierczak-Wojtaś, 2021), the prevalence rate of orthorexia nervosa has been reported to range from 6.9% to 90.6% [sic] using ORTO-15. The recent systematic review and meta-analysis, including 30,476 individuals from 18 countries (López-Gil et al., 2023), demonstrated that the overall proportion of orthorexia nervosa symptoms (assessed using the ORTO-15 with a cut-off of <35) was 27.5%. This means that approximately 3 out of 10 study participants had orthorexia nervosa symptoms, according to the ORTO-15. However, these findings should be interpreted cautiously, considering that only 17.6% of the studies using a cut-off of <35 included representative samples (López-Gil et al., 2023). The overwhelming scientific consensus is that the use of the ORTO-15 to investigate the prevalence of orthorexia nervosa is questionable due to an excessive percentage of falsely positive results in the studied groups. Therefore, these findings need to be interpreted with caution. In addition, it is doubtful whether it describes the current state of affairs. Nevertheless, it is conceivable that the high prevalence of orthorexia nervosa reflects real problems and a willingness to over-report the relevant symptoms, which, in contrast to eating disorders, may be regarded as covetable (Hafstad et al., 2023).

The Düsseldorf Orthorexia Scale seems to be a promising tool for assessing the prevalence of orthorexia nervosa. Prevalence rates using this instrument are substantially lower than other assessment tools (Depa et al., 2017). The prevalence of orthorexia nervosa in the general population has been estimated to range from 0% (e.g. individuals with frequent consumption of meat in Germany) to 28.5% (an adult population in Italy), and in the clinical population, it has been estimated to vary from 0% (e.g. inpatients with somatoform disorders in Germany) to 22.2% (patients with cancer in Lebanon) (Table 7.1).

Table 7.1 Prevalence of orthorexia nervosa using the Düsseldorf Orthorexia Scale in the studies reported in English

| Author(s) and year (in alphabetical order) | Country | Sample | Presence of orthorexia nervosa (≥30 points) | At risk of orthorexia nervosa (25–29 points) |
|---|---|---|---|---|
| Aloi et al., 2023 | Italy | 521 individuals from the general population | 7.5% | 12.9% |
| Barthels et al., 2017 | Germany | 29 inpatients with anorexia nervosa | Nearly all patients reached high scores around the 30-point cut-off* | N/A |
| Barthels et al., 2018 | Germany | 114 individuals following a vegan diet | 7.9% | N/A |
| | | 63 individuals following a vegetarian diet | 3.8% | |
| | | 83 individuals having rare meat consumption | 3.6% | |
| | | 91 individuals having frequent meat consumption | 0% | |
| Barthels et al., 2021 | Germany | 31 patients with somatoform disorders | 6.6% | N/A |
| | | 30 healthy adults | 0% | |
| Brytek-Matera et al., 2020a | Poland Spain | 375 university students from Poland and 485 university students from Spain | 2.6% | 7.9% |
| Brytek-Matera et al., 2020b | Poland | 743 adults | 2.6% | 7.0% |
| | Lebanon | 519 adults | 8.4% | 17.5% |
| Brytek-Matera et al., 2020c | Poland | 229 adults | 3.0% | 5.7% |

**Table 7.1 (cont.)**

| Author(s) and year (in alphabetical order) | Country | Sample | Presence of orthorexia nervosa (≥ 30 points) | | At risk of orthorexia nervosa (25–29 points) |
|---|---|---|---|---|---|
| | | | Admission | Discharge | |
| Brytek-Matera, 2021b | Poland | 412 university students | 6.6% | | 11.9% |
| Cerolini et al., 2022 | Italy | 422 university students | 3.2% | | 4.9% |
| Chard et al., 2019 | United States | 384 undergraduate students | 8.0% | | 12.4% |
| Cosentino et al., 2023 | Italy | 44 patients with type 1 diabetes | 4.5% | | N/A |
| | | 44 healthy adults | 0% | | |
| Depa et al., 2017 | Germany | 456 students | 3.3% | | 9.0% |
| Ferreira and Coimbra, 2021 | Portugal | 513 adults | 10.52% | | 15.01% |
| Greetfeld et al., 2021 | Germany | 511 adults | 2.3% | | 4.9% |
| Greville-Harris et al., 2022 | United Kingdom | 362 adults | N/A | | 38.95% |
| Hallit et al., 2022 | Lebanon | 487 adults | 10.3% | | 23.0% |
| He et al., 2019 | China | 1,075 university students | 7.8% | | 18.2% |
| He et al., 2021 | China | 313 elderly people | 19.5% | | N/A |
| Hessler-Kaufmann et al., 2021 | Germany | Clinical samples | Admission | Discharge | N/A |
| | | 315 inpatients with recurrent depressive disorder | 3.2% | 1.1% | |
| | | 218 inpatients with anorexia nervosa | 48% | 11% | |
| | | 228 inpatients with depressive episode | 1.3% | 2.3% | |
| | | 152 inpatients with obsessive-compulsive disorder | 2.0% | 3.7% | |
| | | 78 inpatients with trauma-related disorders | 1.3% | 0% | |
| | | 63 inpatients with bulimia nervosa | 33% | 7.3% | |
| | | 60 inpatients with phobic disorders | 0% | 2.9% | |
| | | 53 inpatients with somatoform disorders | 0% | 0% | |

**Table 7.1 (cont.)**

| Author(s) and year (in alphabetical order) | Country | Sample | Presence of orthorexia nervosa (≥ 30 points) | At risk of orthorexia nervosa (25–29 points) |
|---|---|---|---|---|
| Lasson et al., 2021; Lasson and Raynal, 2021 | France | 3235 university students | 3.28% | 11.31% |
| Luck-Sikorski et al., 2019 | Germany | 1,007 adults | 6.9% | N/A |
| Parra-Fernández et al., 2019 | Spain | 492 students | 10.5% | N/A |
| Raynal et al., 2022 | France | 441 premenopausal women | 2.7% | 10.2% |
| | | 94 perimenopausal women | 6.4% | 14.9% |
| | | 174 postmenopausal women | 4.6% | 20.7% |
| Rudolph, 2018 | Germany | 1,008 members of fitness clubs | 4.3% | 8.8% |
| Strahler et al., 2018 | Germany | 713 adults | 3.8% | N/A |
| Strahler et al., 2020 | Germany | 391 adults | 4.9% | 13.3% |
| | Lebanon | 519 adults | 8.4% | 17.5% |
| Stutts, 2020 | United States | 217 adults | 9.7% | 11.5% |
| Tarsitano et al., 2022 | Italy | 4,107 adults | 28.5% | N/A |
| Zoghbi et al., 2023 | Lebanon | 366 patients with cancer | 22.2% | 9.0% |

Note: * The DOS does not seem to be able to make a distinction between anorexia nervosa and orthorexia nervosa (Barthels et al., 2017).

Less than half of 1% of college students in the United States of America displayed orthorexia nervosa (Dunn et al., 2016) based on Moroze et al. (2015) criteria for orthorexia nervosa. Despite numerous studies, there are still no reliable data regarding the prevalence of orthorexia nervosa.

# Highlights

• Various questionnaires are used for evaluating orthorexia nervosa. The most common measures used to assess this construct are the ORTO-15, the Eating Habits Questionnaire and the Düsseldorf Orthorexia Scale (tools developed before the publication of the diagnostic criteria by Dunn and Bratman, 2016). The ORTO-15 is the most popular and, simultaneously, the most frequently criticised questionnaire. A key finding of the previous systematic review on psychometric properties of orthorexia nervosa measures was that utilising the ORTO-15 for the assessment of orthorexia nervosa 'is discouraged' (Opitz et al., 2020, p.10). It has been argued that the ORTO-15 has an unacceptable model fit, low internal reliability, and medium-sized correlations with the Eating Habits Questionnaire and the Düsseldorf Orthorexia Scale, suggesting that ORTO-15 measures a different construct and/or investigates orthorexia nervosa less precisely (Meule et al., 2020). Moreover, it has been pointed out that the ORTO-15 is likely to be unable to distinguish between healthy eating and pathological-healthy eating (Dunn et al., 2016). Two other questionnaires, namely the Eating Habits Questionnaire and the Düsseldorf Orthorexia Scale, seem to be reliable measures to assess orthorexia nervosa symptomatology; therefore, we should consider using them instead of the ORTO-15 (Brytek-Matera, 2021a).

• Three novel assessment tools, namely the Teruel Orthorexia Scale, the Barcelona Orthorexia Nervosa Scale and the Orthorexia Nervosa Inventory were developed after Dunn and Bratman's publication of the diagnostic criteria in 2016. The Teruel Orthorexia Scale 'broadens the conceptualisation of orthorexia with differentiable dimensions' (Barrada & Roncero, 2018, p. 289) and distinguishes pathological (orthorexia nervosa) from normative healthy eating (healthy orthorexia). The Barcelona Orthorexia Scale was developed based on the diagnostic criteria for orthorexia nervosa (Dunn & Bratman, 2016). In the development of the Barcelona Orthorexia Scale, the developed item pool was validated by an expert panel selected for their expertise in the areas of orthorexia nervosa and/or eating disorders, strengthening the questionnaire's content validity. The Orthorexia Nervosa Inventory is the first and only assessment measure for orthorexia nervosa, including items about all diagnostic criteria (namely, behaviour and preoccupation with healthy eating, emotional distress, and physical and psychosocial impairment). Both the Barcelona Orthorexia Scale and the Orthorexia Nervosa Inventory require the assessment of their psychometric properties in future studies. The psychometric properties of the novel assessment tools for orthorexia nervosa are promising.

• The recent systematic review and meta-analysis of the association between orthorexia nervosa and obsessive-compulsive symptoms (Huynh et al., 2023) found a significant difference between relationship significance and strength when comparing the first assessment tools for orthorexia nervosa (the ORTO-15, the Eating Habits Questionnaire) to novel assessment tools for orthorexia nervosa (the Düsseldorf Orthorexia Scale, the Orthorexia Nervosa Inventory, the Teruel Orthorexia Scale). By comparison with the first assessment tools that revealed weak (if at all statistically significant) associations (25 studies), novel assessment tools consistently exhibited significant, moderate to strong associations of orthorexia nervosa with obsessive-compulsive symptoms (6 studies).

• Recently, a new revised version of the ORTO-15, the ORTO-R has been proposed. It contains 6 of the previous 15 items of the ORTO-15 and is characterised by better psychometric properties. However, more evidence is needed to examine the reliability and validity of the ORTO-R.

• Despite several measures available, there is still a lack of universal tools for the assessment of orthorexia nervosa and for its diagnosis. The previous systematic review on psychometric properties of quantitative measures assessing orthorexia nervosa (Opitz et al., 2020) revealed that some instruments have either questionable psychometric properties (e.g. the ORTO-15), challenge preliminary diagnostic criteria (e.g. the Düsseldorf Orthorexia Scale) or require further evaluation (e.g. the Orthorexia Nervosa Scale). Additionally, the lack of exhaustive reliability analyses in slightly more than 51% of identified studies suggests that prevalence rates of orthorexia nervosa and its risk assessments could be highly affected by measurement errors (Opitz et al., 2020).

• The prevalence of orthorexia nervosa in the general population as measured by the ORTO-15 was assessed primarily in European studies (Niedzielski & Kaźmierczak-Wojtaś, 2021). The prevalence estimates based on the ORTO-15 have been found to be inflated (unrealistically high) and very different across the samples; thus, they should be considered very carefully (Dunn et al., 2016). Orthorexia nervosa prevalence risk using the Orthorexia Nervosa Inventory among US adults was found to be 4.5% (Oberle, De Nadai & Madrid, 2021), while the prevalence of orthorexia nervosa based on Moroze et al. (2015) criteria was less than 1% (Dunn et al., 2016). The prevalence estimates based on the Düsseldorf Orthorexia Scale ranged from 0% to 28.5% in the general population and from 0% to 22.2% in the clinical population (see Table 7.1). Future studies need to focus on the development of standardising assessment instruments for the diagnosis of orthorexia nervosa. Moreover, priority should be given to epidemiological studies that tend to assess the prevalence of orthorexia nervosa, as well as to longitudinal studies that tend to determine and monitor how the prevalence of orthorexia nervosa changes over time.

# Part IV

# Multidimensional Characteristics of Orthorexia Nervosa

# 8  Psychological Characteristics of Orthorexia Nervosa

## 8.1 Self-Esteem

Self-esteem is a global, one-dimensional and relatively stable construct regarding a positive or negative judgment towards oneself (Rosenberg, 1965). There is evidence that low self-esteem is associated with unhealthy eating behaviours. The recent meta-analysis of longitudinal studies (Krauss et al., 2023), including data from more than 19,000 participants, has found that self-esteem negatively predicted total eating pathology over time and total eating pathology negatively predicted self-esteem over time. It has been suggested that increased self-esteem regarding adherence to the diet characterises individuals with orthorexia nervosa (Bratman & Knight, 2000). Therefore, it is essential to know if this factor might influence the development of orthorexia nervosa. Thus far, few studies have focused on the relationship between orthorexia nervosa and self-esteem. Moreover, there are contradictory results (Table 8.1). Self-esteem was found generally to be unrelated to orthorexia nervosa among university students of health education in Turkey (Özenoğlu & Ünal, 2015), adults in Australia (Barnes & Caltabiano, 2017), adults in Turkey (Yılmaz & Dundar, 2022), and college students in the United States of America (Oberle, Samaghabadi & Hughes, 2017). However, two studies have found that both higher trait self-esteem (Haddad et al., 2019) and higher state self-esteem (Sfeir et al., 2022) were linked to lower levels of orthorexia nervosa in a representative sample of the Lebanese population. Another study has also demonstrated that having high self-esteem reduces the tendency to healthy eating obsession (Yılmaz & Dundar, 2022).

However, it has been reported that individuals with orthorexia nervosa have higher self-esteem than those without orthorexia nervosa and that self-esteem may be positively affected by the self-determined healthy diet (Barnes & Caltabiano, 2017). Thus, they may feel a sense of superiority over others based on their self-determined healthy dietary practices resulting from self-discipline, perfectionism and individual responsibility (Bratman & Knight, 2000), and striving for a perfect diet may result in high self-esteem, as those who follow it may feel virtuous due to their self-determined healthy eating behaviours (Musolino et al., 2015). In addition, individuals with orthorexia nervosa may believe that they can make healthy food choices to provide for their health

**Table 8.1** The summary of existing (cross-sectional) studies examining the relationship between orthorexia nervosa and self-esteem among adults

| Author(s) and year | Measurement of orthorexia nervosa | Measurement of self-esteem | Sample | Results: relationship between orthorexia nervosa and self-esteem | | |
| --- | --- | --- | --- | --- | --- | --- |
| | | | | Positive association | Negative association | Lack of association |
| Özenoğlu and Ünal, 2015 | ORTO-11 | The Coopersmith Self-Esteem Inventory | 165 students (127 women) $M_{age} = 20.37 \pm 1.75$ years | | | ✓ |
| Barnes and Caltabiano, 2017 | ORTO-15 | The Rosenberg Self-Esteem Scale | 220 adults (174 women) $M_{age} = 23.81 \pm 8.40$ years | | | ✓ |
| Oberle, Samaghabadi and Hughes, 2017 | The Eating Habits Questionnaire | The Rosenberg Self-Esteem Scale | 459 undergraduate students (371 women) N/A | | | ✓ |
| Haddad et al., 2019 | ORTO-15 | The Rosenberg Self-Esteem Scale | 806 adults (536 women) $M_{age} = 27.59 \pm 11.76$ years | ✓ $r = 0.084$ $p = 0.019$ | | |
| Sfeir et al., 2022 | The Teruel Orthorexia Scale | The Rosenberg Self-Esteem Scale The State Self-Esteem Scale | 428 adults (283 women) $M_{age} = 23.57 \pm 7.38$ years | | ✓ $r = -0.27$ $p < 0.001$ (state self-esteem) | ✓ (trait self-esteem) |
| Yilmaz and Dundar, 2022 | ORTO-11 | The Rosenberg Self-Esteem Scale | 248 adults (104 women) $M_{age} = 42.6 \pm 6.3$ years | | | ✓ |

(Brytek-Matera et al., 2019) and that can also lead to a higher sense of self-worth. There are also studies considering low self-esteem to be a predisposing factor for orthorexia nervosa (Bóna, Erdész & Túry, 2021; Yılmaz & Dundar, 2022). Nevertheless, based on the existing findings, it cannot be concluded that self-esteem seems to be strongly connected to orthorexia nervosa, unlike eating disorders (Krauss et al., 2023). In addition, the previous review on psychosocial risk factors of orthorexia nervosa (McComb & Mills, 2019) has not identified self-esteem as a determinant that contributes to the onset of orthorexia nervosa. It has been suggested that this was because of the few existing studies that included self-esteem as a possible determinant factor. Therefore, no definitive conclusions can be drawn at this point. The evidence base for self-esteem and its relationship with orthorexia nervosa is limited to date, and further research is needed to examine its potential to alter this inappropriate eating behaviour.

## 8.2 Personality Traits

Up to now, a limited number of studies have examined the relationship of orthorexia nervosa with factors that have been previously implicated in anorexia nervosa and/or obsessive-compulsive disorder. Research on the personality correlates of orthorexia nervosa revealed that increased orthorexia nervosa symptomatology is associated with higher levels of perfectionism (e.g. Barnes & Caltabiano, 2017; Oberle, Samaghabadi & Hughes, 2017), neuroticism (Gleaves et al., 2013; Strahler et al., 2020), narcissism (Oberle, Samaghabadi & Hughes, 2017; Brunett & Oberle, 2022), negative affectivity (Strahler et al., 2020), psychoticism (Award et al., 2022; Roncero et al., 2021; Strahler et al., 2020), Machiavellianism (Brunett & Oberle, 2022) and psychopathy (Brunett & Oberle, 2022) (Table 8.2).

Orthorexia nervosa was found to be predicted by two personality factors: negative affectivity (characterised by difficulty in regulating emotions and negative affect) and psychoticism (characterised by eccentricity, feeling special and holding beliefs outside the norm) (Roncero et al., 2021). It has also been demonstrated that high harm avoidance (characterised by excessive worrying, pessimism and shyness), low self-directedness (ability to regulate behaviour to achieve personal goals) and higher transcendence (associated with spiritual experiences and transpersonal identification) characterised individuals with a high risk of orthorexia nervosa compared to those with a low risk of orthorexia nervosa (Kiss-Leizer & Rigó, 2019). The 'orthorexic personality' was described as marked 'by excessive worrying, along with being fearful and anxious, which is manifested by shyness in social situations, matched with the desire to be perfect and accepted' (Kiss-Leizer & Rigó, 2019, p. 33).

**Table 8.2** The examples of (cross-sectional) studies examining the relationship between orthorexia nervosa and personality traits among adults

| Author(s) and year | Measurement of orthorexia nervosa | Measurement of personality | Sample | Results: relationship between orthorexia nervosa and personality traits | | |
|---|---|---|---|---|---|---|
| | | | | Problems | Knowledge | Feelings |
| Gleaves et al., 2013 | The Eating Habits Questionnaire | The Personality Assessment Screener | 213 undergraduate students (65% women) $Mage = 20.00\pm2.64$ years | Negative affect | | |
| | | International | | $r = 0.25^{**}$ | $r = 0.17^{*}$ | $r = 0.18^{*}$ |
| | | - Negative affect | | Alcohol Problems | | |
| | | - Acting out | | $r = 0.20^{**}$ | $r = 0.14^{*}$ | - |
| | | - Health problems | | | Conscientiousness | |
| | | - Psychotic features | | | | |
| | | - Social withdrawal | | Neuroticism | $r = 0.17^{*}$ | $r = 0.20^{**}$ |
| | | - Hostile control | | $r = 0.31^{**}$ | - | $r = 0.19^{**}$ |
| | | - Suicidal thinking | | Health problems | | Extraversion |
| | | - Alienation | | $r = 0.18^{*}$ | | $r = 0.15^{*}$ |
| | | - Alcohol problem | | Suicidal thinking | | |
| | | - Anger control | | $r = 0.14^{*}$ | | |
| | | The Personality Item Pool Five Factor Personality Inventory | | | | |
| | | - Openness | | | | |
| | | - Conscientiousness | | | | |
| | | - Extraversion | | | | |
| | | - Agreeableness | | | | |
| | | - Neuroticism | | | | |

Table 8.2 (cont.– Part A)

| Author(s) and year | Measurement of orthorexia nervosa | Measurement of personality | Sample | Results: relationship between orthorexia nervosa and personality traits | | |
|---|---|---|---|---|---|---|
| | | | | Problems | Behaviours | Feelings |
| Oberle, Samaghabadi & Hughes, 2017 | The Eating Habits Questionnaire | The Narcissistic Personality Inventory | 459 students (80.8% women) $M_{age}$ =19.85±2.79 years | Narcissism | $r = 0.18^{**}$ | $r = 0.11^{*}$ |
| | | The Frost Multidimensional Perfectionism Scale- Personal standards | | Personal standards $r = 0.11^{*}$ | $r = 0.25^{***}$ | $r = 0.20^{***}$ |
| | | – Organisation | | Organisation $r = 0.25^{***}$ | $r = 0.11^{*}$ | $r = 0.20^{***}$ |
| | | – Concern over mistakes | | Concern over mistakes $r = 0.13^{*}$ | | |
| | | – Doubts about actions | | Doubts about actions $r = 0.23^{***}$ | | |
| | | – Parental expectations | | Parental criticism $r = 0.18^{***}$ | | |
| | | – Parental criticism | | Parental expectation $r = 0.20^{***}$ | | |
| | | | | $r = 0.21^{***}$ | | |
| Barnes and Caltabiano, 2017 | The ORTO-15° | The Multidimensional Perfectionism Scale | 220 adults (174 women) $M_{age}$ = 23.81±8.40 years | Self-oriented perfectionism: $r = -0.365^{**}$ | | |
| | | – Self-oriented perfectionism | | Others-oriented perfectionism: $r = -0.250^{**}$ | | |
| | | – Others-oriented perfectionism | | Socially prescribed perfectionism: $r = -0.238^{**}$ | | |
| | | – Socially prescribed perfectionism | | | | |

**Table 8.2 (cont.– Part B)**

| Author(s) and year | Measurement of orthorexia nervosa | Measurement of personality | Sample | Results: relationship between orthorexia nervosa and personality traits | |
|---|---|---|---|---|---|
| | | | | German adults | Lebanese adults |
| Strahler et al., 2020 | The Düsseldorf Orthorexia Scale (DOS) | The Big Five Inventory | 519 adults (56% women) | Agreeableness | |
| | The Teruel Orthorexia Scale (TOS-ON^) | - Extraversion | $M_{age}$ =36.02 ± 14.20 years | TOS-ON: $r = -0.108$* | DOS: $r = -0.098$* |
| | | - Agreeableness | | | TOS-ON: $r = -0.253$*** |
| | | - Conscientiousness | | Neuroticism | |
| | | - Neuroticism | | DOS: $r = 0.228$*** | TOS-ON: $r = 0.106$* |
| | | - Openness | | TOS-ON: $r = 0.319$*** | |
| | | The Personality Inventory for the Diagnostic and Statistical Manual of Mental Disorders 5th Edition (PID–5–BF) –Adult (brief form) | | Extraversion | DOS: $r = -0.098$* |
| | | - Negative affectivity | | Openness | |
| | | - Detachment | | | DOS: $r = -0.095$* |
| | | - Antagonism | | TOS-ON: | |
| | | - Disinhibition | | $r = -0.191$*** | |
| | | - Psychoticism | | Conscientiousness | |
| | | | | | DOS: $r = -0.187$*** |

Table 8.2 (cont.– Part C)

| Author(s) and year | Measurement of orthorexia nervosa | Measurement of personality | Sample | Results: relationship between orthorexia nervosa and personality traits |
|---|---|---|---|---|
| | | | | Negative affectivity |
| | | | | DOS: r = 0.184*** DOS: r = −0.096* |
| | | | | TOS-ON: |
| | | | | r = 0.298*** |
| | | | | Detachment |
| | | | | DOS: r = 0.191*** TOS-ON: |
| | | | | TOS-ON: r = 0.094* |
| | | | | r = 0.258*** |
| | | | | Antagonism |
| | | | | TOS-ON: TOS-ON: |
| | | | | r = 0.203*** r = 0.146*** |
| | | | | Psychoticism |
| | | | | DOS: r = 0.199*** TOS-ON: |
| | | | | TOS-ON: r = 0.111** |
| | | | | r = 0.305*** |
| | | | | Disinhibition |
| | | | | DOS: r = 0.130** |
| | | | | TOS-ON: |
| | | | | r = 0.239*** |

Table 8.2 (cont.– Part D)

| Author(s) and year | Measurement of orthorexia nervosa | Measurement of personality | Sample | Results: relationship between orthorexia nervosa and personality traits |
|---|---|---|---|---|
| Roncero et al., 2021 | The Teruel Orthorexia Scale (TOS-ON^) | The Personality Inventory for DSM-5 – Short Form (see Strahler et al., 2020 in this Table) | 297 adults (94.6% women) $M_{age}$ =30.08 ± 12.90 years | Negative affectivity: $r = 0.36*$ Detachment: $r = 0.23*$ Disinhibition: $r = 0.21*$ Psychoticism: $r = 0.26*$ |
| Award et al., 2022 | The Teruel Orthorexia Scale (TOS-ON^) | for the Diagnostic and Statistical Manual of Mental Disorders 5th Edition (PID–5–BF) –Adult (brief form) (see Strahler et al., 2020 in this Table) The I–8 (measured impulsivity) - Urgency - Premeditation - Perseverance - Sensation seeking | 519 adults (56% women) $M_{age}$ =27.59 ± 11.76 years | Detachment: $r = 0.126**$ Antagonism: $r = 0.176***$ Psychoticism: $r = 0.152**$ Urgency: $r = 0.125**$ Premeditation: $r = 0.110*$ Perseverance: $r = 0.169***$ Sensation seeking: $r = -0.111***$ |
| Brunett & Oberle, 2022 | The Orthorexia Nervosa Inventory | The Short Dark Triad Scale - Machiavellianism - Narcissism - Psychopathy | 788 adults (74% women) N/A | Machiavellianism: $r = 0.42**$ Narcissism: $r = 0.11**$ Psychopathy: $r = 0.51**$ |

Note: ˄ In ORTO-11 and ORTO-15, a score of 1 is attributed to responses that are more indicative of orthorexia nervosa, whereas a score of 4 is given to those that indicate normal eating behaviour. Therefore, lower scores correspond to more pathological behaviour.

^TOS-ON: Orthorexia nervosa. Healthy orthorexia was not presented in this Table due to its 'normative' eating behaviour.

$*p < 0.05$ $**p < 0.01$. $***p < 0.001$.

The previous study also highlighted that perfectionism was indirectly and positively linked to orthorexia nervosa symptoms via a health-focused self-concept in individuals high in erroneous beliefs (Yung & Tabri, 2022). In addition, a health-focused self-concept was indirectly and positively associated with symptoms of orthorexia nervosa via fear and disgust in individuals who believed they were currently following a healthy eating diet plan and/or believed they were leading a healthy eating lifestyle (Tabri, Yung & Elliott, 2022).

It has also been found that individuals with high orthorexic tendencies demonstrate higher levels of different facets of perfectionism, namely perfectionistic strivings (which refers to high personal standards and self-oriented pursuit of perfection) and perfectionistic concerns (which regard concerns about mistakes, fear of negative evaluations from others to not being perfect, and adverse reactions to imperfection) as well as perfectionism linked to obsessive-compulsive features and characteristics of eating disorders in comparison with individuals with low orthorexic tendencies (Novara et al., 2023). It has been suggested that perfectionism, a common feature between eating disorders, obsessive-compulsive disorder and orthorexia nervosa, can be considered a transdiagnostic process (central to the psychopathology of eating disorders and obsessive-compulsive disorder) in orthorexia nervosa as well (Novara et al., 2023).

## 8.3 Eating Behaviours

### 8.3.1 Disordered Eating Behaviours

Orthorexia nervosa seems to be closely related to eating disorder behaviours (Atchison & Zickgraf, 2022). This link is complex and still far from being thoroughly understood. When looking into the relationship between orthorexia nervosa and disordered eating, results are inconclusive: numerous research has found that higher levels of disordered eating behaviours (i.e. dieting, bulimia and oral control) are associated with higher levels of orthorexia nervosa (e.g. Asil & Sürücüoğlu, 2015; Caferoglu & Toklu, 2022; Gonidakis et al., 2021; Kaya et al., 2022; Parra-Fernández et al., 2021; Roncero et al., 2017). Some reported that lower levels of orthorexia nervosa were linked to higher levels of disordered eating behaviours (Brytek-Matera et al., 2017; Hallit, Brytek-Matera & Obeid, 2021), while others indicated a lack of the relationship between orthorexia nervosa and disordered eating behaviour among women (Brytek-Matera et al., 2017) (Table 8.3).

Some studies have suggested that orthorexia nervosa is unrelated to emotional eating (Brytek-Matera et al., 2019; Grammatikopoulou et al., 2018; He et al., 2019; Strahler et al., 2018), others have found evidence of its positive association

**Table 8.3** The summary of existing (cross-sectional) studies examining the relationship between orthorexia nervosa and disordered eating behaviour among adults

| Author(s) and year | Measurement of orthorexia nervosa | Measurement of disordered eating behaviour | Sample | Results of the association between orthorexia nervosa and disordered eating behaviour |
|---|---|---|---|---|
| Asil and Sürücüoğlu, 2015 | ORTO-15* | The Eating Attitudes Test–40 | 117 Turkish dietitians (86.3% women) $M_{age} = 34 \pm 11.2$ years | $r_{EAT-26\ total\ score} = -0.307; p = 0.001$ |
| Aiello et al., 2022 | The ORTO-15* | The Eating Attitudes Test–26 The Starvation Symptom Inventory | 160 Italian and Spanish university students (∅**) | $r_{EAT-26\ total\ score} = -0.363; p < 0.001$ $r_{Dieting} = -0.429; p < 0.001$ $r_{Bulimia} = -0.188; p < 0.001$ $r_{Starvation\ symptoms} = -0.169; p < 0.05$ |
| Brytek-Matera et al., 2014 | The ORTO-15* | The Eating Attitudes Test–26 | 400 Polish university students (85.25% women) Women $M_{age} = 23.09 \pm 3.14$ years Men $M_{age} = 24.02 \pm 3.87$ years | Factor 1 $r_{EAT-26\ total\ score} = -0.28; p < 0.001$ $r_{Dieting} = -0.36; p < 0.001$ $r_{Bulimia} = -0.07; p > 0.05$ $r_{Oral\ control} = -0.01; p > 0.05$ Factor 2 $r_{EAT-26\ total\ score} = -0.65; p < 0.001$ $r_{Dieting} = -0.59; p < 0.001$ $r_{Bulimia} = -0.67; p < 0.001$ $r_{Oral\ control} = -0.23; p < 0.001$ |

**Table 8.3 (cont. – Part A)**

| Author(s) and year | Measurement of orthorexia nervosa | Measurement of disordered eating behaviour | Sample | Results of the association between orthorexia nervosa and disordered eating behaviour |
|---|---|---|---|---|
| Brytek-Matera et al., 2017 | The ORTO-15* | The Eating Attitudes Test–26 | 120 Italian university students (69.16% women) $M_{age} = 22.74 \pm 7.31$ years | Women $r_{EAT-26\ total\ score} = 0.01; p > 0.05$ Men $r_{EAT-26\ total\ score} = 0.35; p < 0.05$ |
| Bundros et al., 2016 | The Bratman Orthorexia Test | The Eating Attitudes Test–26 | 448 American college students (? women) $M_{age} = 22.00 \pm ?$ years | $r_{EAT-26\ total\ score} = 0.47; p < 0.01$ |
| Caferoglu and Toklu, 2022 | ORTO-11* | The Eating Attitudes Test–26 | 1,429 Turkish dietitians and dietetic students (90.8% women) $M_{age} = 23.20 \pm 4.88$ years | |
| Falgares et al., 2023 | The Teruel Orthorexia Scale | The Eating Disorder Inventory – third edition | 782 Italian adults (82% female) $M_{age} = 32.3 \pm 11.55$ years | $r_{Orthorexia\ nervosa} = 0.68; p < 0.001$ $r_{Healthy\ orthorexia} = -0.02; p > 0.05$ |
| Freire et al., 2020 | The ORTO-15* | The Eating Attitudes Test–26 | 60 Brazilian exercise practitioners (63.33% women) $M_{age} = 28.58 \pm 7.76$ years | $r_{EAT-26\ total\ score} = -0.42; p < 0.05$ |
| Gorrasi et al., 2020 | The ORTO-15* | The Eating Attitudes Test–26 | 918 Italian students (54.8% women) $M_{age} = 20.2 \pm 1.7$ years | $r_{EAT-26\ total\ score} = -0.282$ $p < 0.001$ |
| Gorrasi et al., 2022 | The ORTO-15* | The Eating Attitudes Test–26 | Web-based survey (WBS): 137 Italian students (61.3% women) $M_{age} = 20.4 \pm 2.8$ years Paper-based survey (PBS): 372 Italian students (57% women) $M_{age} = 20.0 \pm 1.3$ years | WBS $r_{EAT-26\ total\ score} = -0.362$ $p < 0.001$ PBS $r_{EAT-26\ total\ score} = -0.307$ $p < 0.001$ |

**Table 8.3 (cont.– Part B)**

| Author(s) and year | Measurement of orthorexia nervosa | Measurement of disordered eating behaviour | Sample | Results of the association between orthorexia nervosa and disordered eating behaviour |
|---|---|---|---|---|
| Hallit et al., 2021 | The ORTO-R | The Eating Attitudes Test–26 | 783 Lebanese adults (33.5% women) $M_{age} = 27.78 \pm 11.60$ years | Women $r_{EAT-26\ total\ score} = 0.428; p < 0.001$ $r_{Dieting} = 0.501; p < 0.001$ $r_{Bulimia} = 0.262; p < 0.001$ $r_{Oral\ control} = 0.226; p < 0.001$ Men $r_{EAT-26\ total\ score} = 0.360; p < 0.001$ $r_{Dieting} = 0.423; p < 0.001$ $r_{Bulimia} = 0.232; p < 0.001$ $r_{Oral\ control} = 0.279; p < 0.001$ |
| Kaya, Uzdil and Çakıroğlu (2022) | The Orthorexia Nervosa Inventory | The Eating Attitudes Test–26 | 710 Turkish adults (70.8% women) $M_{age} = 30.15 \pm 7.47$ years | $r_{Total\ score} = 0.418; p < 0.01$ $r_{Behaviours} = 0.311; p < 0.01$ $r_{Impairments} = 0.374; p < 0.05$ $r_{Emotions} = 0.401; p < 0.05$ |
| Mitrofanova et al., 2021 | The ORTO-15* | The Eating Attitudes Test–26 | 50 British adults (60% women) $M_{age} = 34.0 \pm 14.4$ years | $r_{EAT-26\ total\ score} = -0.66$ $p < 0.001$ |
| Oberle, De Nadai and Madrid, 2021 | The Orthorexia Nervosa Inventory | The Eating Attitudes Test–26 | 847 American adults (82% women) $M_{age} = 21.72 \pm 6.74$ years | $r_{Total\ score} = 0.79; p < 0.001$ $r_{Behaviours} = 0.59; p < 0.001$ $r_{Impairments} = 0.72; p < 0.001$ $r_{Emotions} = 0.81; p < 0.001$ |

**Table 8.3 (cont.– Part C)**

| Author(s) and year | Measurement of orthorexia nervosa | Measurement of disordered eating behaviour | Sample | Results of the association between orthorexia nervosa and disordered eating behaviour |
|---|---|---|---|---|
| Parra-Fernández et al., 2021 | The Eating Habits Questionnaire | The Eating Attitudes Test–26 | 487 Spanish university students:<br>Sample 1 ($N_1$) = 286 (81.9% women)<br>Sample 2 ($N_2$) = 201 (52.2% women)<br>$N_1 M_{age}$ = 21.75 ± 5.10 years<br>$N_2 M_{age}$ = 21.17 ± 6.81 years | **Knowledge of healthy eating**<br>$r_{EAT-26\ total\ score}$ = 0.391; $p < 0.01$<br>$r_{Dieting}$ = 0.515; $p < 0.01$<br>$r_{Bulimia}$ = 0.379; $p < 0.01$<br>$r_{Worry\ about\ food}$ = 0.242; $p < 0.01$<br>$r_{Oral\ control}$ = 0.084; $p > 0.05$<br>**Problems associated with healthy eating**<br>$r_{EAT-26\ total\ score}$ = 0.629; $p < 0.01$<br>$r_{Dieting}$ = 0.595; $p < 0.01$<br>$r_{Bulimia}$ = 0.645; $p < 0.01$<br>$r_{Worry\ about\ food}$ = 0.488; $p < 0.01$<br>$r_{Oral\ control}$ = 0.257 ; $p < 0.01$<br>**Feeling positively about healthy eating**<br>$r_{EAT-26\ total\ score}$ = 0.459; $p < 0.01$<br>$r_{Dieting}$ = 0.537; $p < 0.01$<br>$r_{Bulimia}$ = 0.398; $p < 0.01$<br>$r_{Worry\ about\ food}$ = 0.050; $p < 0.01$<br>$r_{Oral\ control}$ = 1.16 ; $p > 0.05$ |
| Rogowska et al., 2021 | The Test of Orthorexia Nervosa (TON-17) | The Eating Attitudes Test–26 | 767 Polish adults (56.98% women)<br>$M_{age}$ = 26.49 ± 9.66 years | $r_{EAT-26\ total\ score}$ = 0.36<br>$p < 0.001$ |

**Table 8.3 (cont.– Part D)**

| Author(s) and year | Measurement of orthorexia nervosa | Measurement of disordered eating behaviour | Sample | Results of the association between orthorexia nervosa and disordered eating behaviour |
|---|---|---|---|---|
| Roncero, Barrada and Perpiñá, 2017 | The ORTO-15** | The Eating Attitudes Test–26<br><br>Self-Report Yale-Brown Cornell Eating Disorders Scale | 242 Spanish university students (63.2% women)<br><br>$M_{age} = 24.94 \pm 7.07$ years | $r_{Dieting} = -0.59; p < 0.05$<br>$r_{Bulimia} = -0.67; p < 0.05$<br>$r_{Oral\,control} = -0.23; p < 0.05$<br>$r_{Preoccupations} = 0.23; p < 0.05$<br>$r_{Rituals} = 0.29; p < 0.05$<br>$r_{Severity\,Preoccupations} = 0.06; p > 0.05$<br>$r_{Severity\,rituals} = 0.10; p > 0.05$ |
| Souza et al., 2021 | The Düsseldorf Orthorexia Scale | The Eating Attitudes Test–26 | 486 Brazilian dietitians and college students (60% women)<br><br>$M_{age} = 27$ years | $r_{EAT-26\,total\,score} = 0.488$<br>$p < 0.01$<br><br>$r_{Dieting} = 0.470; p < 0.01$<br>$r_{Bulimia} = 0.468; p < 0.01$<br>$r_{Oral\,control} = 0.115; p > 0.05$ |
| Uriegas et al., 2021 | ORTO-15* | The Eating Attitudes Test–26 | 1,090 American student athletes (69.35% women)<br><br>$M_{age} = 19.6 \pm 1.4$ years | The presence of risk of orthorexia nervosa:<br><br>$Exp\,(B)_{Dieting} = 1.16; p < 0.001$<br>$Exp\,(B)_{Bulimia} = 1.29; p < 0.001$<br>$Exp\,(B)_{Oral\,control} = 1.16; p < 0.001$ |

Note: * In ORTO-11 and ORTO-15, a score of 1 is attributed to responses that are more indicative of orthorexia nervosa, whereas a score of 4 is given to those that indicate normal eating behaviour. Therefore, lower scores correspond to more pathological behaviour. ** Lack of information about the number of women.
*** Contrary to the original scoring of the ORTO-15, higher values correspond to higher orthorexia nervosa.

with emotional eating and uncontrolled eating (Brytek-Matera, Plasonja & Décamps, 2020; Şentürk et al., 2022), while there is also one study (He et al., 2019) demonstrating its negative association with uncontrolled eating.

The previous study (Gramaglia et al., 2019) found that individuals with a high level of concern about dieting are more likely to display orthorexia nervosa than those who do not follow a diet. They score in a range that suggests disordered eating (Dunn et al., 2017). Other research (Gorrassi et al., 2020) demonstrated that participants with orthorexia nervosa are more likely to be on a diet and have a higher prevalence of risk of eating disorders than those without orthorexia nervosa. Dieting was also positively associated with and positively predictive of orthorexia nervosa (Brytek-Matera et al., 2019; Gorrassi et al., 2020; Gramaglia et al., 2019; Reynolds, 2018; Strahler et al., 2018). Perhaps the link between orthorexia nervosa and dieting may be explained by the great attention paid to the individual responsibility for health, according to the foundation of healthism and neoliberalism, viewing health as an individual's responsibility. The association between dieting and orthorexia nervosa has also been proposed to be interpreted in two ways: restricting intake of high-caloric foods and preoccupation with body image and shape can increase the risk of developing orthorexia nervosa or preoccupation with healthy eating can provoke a preoccupation with weight and shape, later seen in other eating disorders (McComb & Mills, 2019). According to some researchers (Novara et al., 2021a), pursuing a diet could represent a prodrome of an eating disorder or an interfering behaviour within the treatment of eating disorders.

Orthorexia nervosa involves disordered eating above and beyond a simple commitment to healthy eating behaviours (Oberle, De Nadai & Madrid, 2021) and should be distinguished from non-problematic forms of interest in healthy eating (Costanzo et al., 2022). Disordered eating attitude (abnormal beliefs, thoughts, feelings, behaviours and relationships regarding food) (Rogowska et al., 2021), self-reported current eating disorder (Gramaglia et al., 2019) and eating disorder features (Brytek-Matera, 2021b; Parra-Fernández et al., 2018a; 2018b; 2019) are related with orthorexia nervosa. It has also been indicated that individuals who report higher levels of orthorexia nervosa are more likely to report higher levels of eating disorder features (Falgares et al., 2023). Some previous studies have demonstrated that orthorexia nervosa involves associations related to dietary restraint, eating concern and cognitive preoccupations about weight and body shape (Strahler et al., 2018; Tremelling et al., 2017), while other research has found that eating concern, weight concern and shape concern have no relationship with orthorexia nervosa (Heiss et al., 2019). Higher levels of pronounced eating disorder pathology have been observed in individuals with orthorexia nervosa than in those without orthorexia nervosa

(Strahler et al., 2018; Tremelling et al., 2017). Individuals with orthorexia nervosa present higher levels of the eating disorder risk composite than the healthy eating control group and normal eating control group (Costanzo et al., 2022). Clinically relevant symptoms of an eating disorder were observed in 77.8% of individuals with orthorexia nervosa compared to 28.9% of those without orthorexia nervosa (Strahler et al., 2018). Individuals with anorexia nervosa and bulimia nervosa, as well as those following the 'zone diet', display higher levels of orthorexia nervosa than those who are not following any diet (Novara et al., 2022a). Recently, a prospective study (Messer, Liu & Linardon, 2023) established that symptoms of orthorexia nervosa prospectively predicted changes in eating disorder psychopathology (an increase in binge eating, driven exercise episodes and eating concerns) and general mental health problems (an increase of depressive symptoms) among a non-clinical sample of adults (Messer, Liu & Linardon, 2023). To sum up, the vast majority of existing studies (see Table 8.3) have indicated that orthorexia nervosa is related to disordered eating behaviours, suggesting the dependency of orthorexia nervosa on problematic eating conditions.

### 8.3.2 Food Addition

Food addiction reflects abnormal eating patterns referred to as excessive consumption of highly processed foods that contain high combinations of sugar, salt and fat (Gearhardt et al., 2009). Food addiction has not been explored yet in orthorexia nervosa. Despite that, there are two studies (Grammatikopoulou et al., 2018; Sultana et al., 2022) combining dietary intake data with the assessment of orthorexia nervosa and food addiction (Table 8.4). A previous study (Sultana et al., 2022) demonstrated that students from Bangladesh are more at risk of food addiction and less so for orthorexia nervosa. In contrast, the results were the opposite for students from Greece (Grammatikopoulou et al., 2018).

### 8.3.3 Mindful Eating

Mindful eating (i.e. paying attention to food on purpose, moment by moment, without judgment) is an approach to food that focuses on individuals' sensual awareness of the food and their experience of the food (Nelson, 2017). In short, it permits awareness of what we eat, why we eat, and how it makes us feel. According to Mantzios (2021: in Miley et al., 2022), 'mindful eating behaviour is defined as the sustained attention on a sensory element of the eating exercise (e.g. the taste), and a non-judgmental (or non-evaluative) awareness of thoughts and feelings that are incongruent to the sensory elements of the present eating experiences' (p. 2870), which is more specific to behaviour itself, rather than decision-making that is co-occurring when eating mindfully (Miley et al.,

Table 8.4 The summary of existing (cross-sectional) studies examining orthorexia nervosa and food addiction among university students

| Author(s) and year | Objective(s) of the study | Sample characteristics | Methods | Results | Conclusion |
|---|---|---|---|---|---|
| Grammati-kopoulou et al., 2018 | • To evaluate stress-related eating, food addiction and orthorexia nervosa in relation to the dietary intake among nutrition/ dietetics students. | Greece; 176 undergraduate students (140 women) aged between 18 and 40 years<br><br>$M_{age} =$ 21.7±1.9;years<br><br>$M_{BMI} =$ 24.06 ± 4.72 kg/m$^2$ | • The Bratman Orthorexia Test<br>• The modi-fied Yale Food Addiction<br>• The Eating and Appraisal Due to Emotion and Stress Questionnaire<br>• a 3-day food diary | • No differences were observed between men and women concerning the prevalence of food addiction and orthorexia nervosa.<br>• Students with orthorexia nervosa exhibited increased body mass index, reduced energy and saturated fat intake in comparison with those without orthorexia nervosa.<br>• Women with orthorexia nervosa exhibited increased body mass index and waist circumference compared to those without orthorexia nervosa.<br>• Men with orthorexia nervosa consumed more vegetables than those without orthorexia nervosa.<br>• Orthorexia nervosa was associated with increased body mass index, waist circumference and energy intake. | • A great number of dietetics students were prone to orthorexia, and a small percentage demonstrated food addiction. |

**Table 8.4 (cont.)**

| Author(s) and year | Objective(s) of the study | Sample characteristics | Methods | Results | Conclusion |
|---|---|---|---|---|---|
| | | | | • Students with food addiction exhibited more emotion- and stress-related eating than those without food addiction.<br><br>• Emotion- and stress-related eating was negatively associated with body mass index. | |
| Sultana et al., 2022 | • To explore the prevalence of orthorexia nervosa and food addiction.<br><br>• To examine the factors associated with orthorexia nervosa, food addiction and dietary diversity during the COVID–19 pandemic. | Convenience sampling technique;<br><br>Bangladesh: 4,076 university students (2236 women) aged between 18 and 28 years<br><br>$M_{age} = 22.07 \pm 1.69$ years | • The Bratman Orthorexia Test<br><br>• The modified Yale Food Addiction Scale<br><br>• The dietary diversity (DD) score<br><br>• The Eating Attitudes Test | • The prevalence of orthorexia nervosa was 1.7%.<br><br>• Participants with orthorexia nervosa consumed more legumes, nuts, seeds, dark green leafy vegetables, vitamin A rich fruits and vegetables, milk and milk products.<br><br>• Older individuals (24–28 years), married, formerly smoked, were of lower socio-economic status, had normal weight, had fitness goals, had lost weight compared to the pre-COVID-19 period, experienced feelings of guilt when violating food rules, and had good problem-solving skills and social interactions were more likely to have orthorexia nervosa. | • Students from Bangladesh are at risk of food addiction, and less so for orthorexia nervosa.<br><br>• Nutritional awareness programmes focusing on dietary diversity and healthy eating habits should be implemented for students. |

Table 8.4 (cont.)

| Author(s) and year | Objective(s) of the study | Sample characteristics | Methods | Results | Conclusion |
|---|---|---|---|---|---|
| | | | | • Individuals who were female, actively smoked, were married, were overweight or obese, had fitness goals, had feelings of guilt consistently when violating food rules, poor social interactions, and weight loss as compared to the pre-COVID-19 period were more likely to have a food addiction.<br><br>• Dietary diversity was associated with older age (24–28 years), being of middle or upper socio-economic status and having fitness goals.<br><br>• The prevalence of food addiction was 7.5%.<br><br>• Participants with food addiction consumed more organ meats and eggs. | • Frequent screening and awareness programmes may help lower risks of disordered eating and their impacts on health and overall well-being among university students. |

2022). The purpose of mindful eating is not to lose weight (although it is highly likely that it may facilitate weight management) but to savour the moment and the food and be fully present for the eating experience (Nelson, 2017).

Mindful eating encourages and promotes healthier weight and eating behaviours (Jordan et al., 2014; Mantzios, Skillett & Egan, 2019), including an increased intake of fruit and vegetables (Timmerman et al., 2017), reductions in high sugar, intake of high-calorie foods and total energy intake (Allirot et al., 2018; Mantzios et al., 2018; Seguias & Tapper, 2018; Winkens et al., 2020), as well as negative mood and food cravings (Sagui-Henson et al., 2021). It may also influence the serving size of energy-dense foods more than daily mindfulness (Beshara et al., 2013). It is worth pointing out that mindfulness affects eating behaviour by encouraging attitudinal preferences for healthier foods (Jordan et al., 2014). Substantial cross-sectional data suggest that higher trait mindfulness is related to healthier food choices and a healthier diet (e.g. Farrar, Plagnol & Tapper, 2022; Sala et al., 2020), more precisely to less impulsive eating, reduced calorie consumption and healthier snack choices. Therefore, generic mindfulness-based strategies could have ancillary benefits for encouraging healthier eating behaviour (Jordan et al., 2014). Mindful eating can potentially address problematic eating behaviours, and mindfulness-based approaches appear most effective in addressing binge eating, emotional eating and eating in response to external cues (Warren et al., 2017).

The previous study (Strahler, 2021) demonstrated that higher mindfulness is linked to healthy orthorexia, whereas lower trait mindfulness is associated with orthorexia nervosa in adults. Some recent studies have looked at the effects of mindful eating on orthorexia nervosa, indicating no association between orthorexia nervosa and mindful eating in individuals following a vegan diet (Kalika, Egan & Mantzios, 2022), positive association between focused eating (a facet of mindful eating) and orthorexia nervosa and negative association between mindful eating (especially eating with awareness; Miley et al., 2022) and orthorexia nervosa in adults (Demirer & Yardımcı, 2024; Kalika et al., 2023; Thorne et al., 2023) (Table 8.5). Therefore, it could be assumed that mindful eating can act as a protective factor in orthorexia nervosa and promote healthier eating in the adult population. This hypothesis needs more in-depth exploration in the future.

## 8.4 Health-Related Beliefs and Behaviours

Given that individuals with orthorexia nervosa are driven by the desire to achieve perfect physical health and the motivation to pursue a healthier lifestyle, the commitment to healthy eating may conceivably extend to their

Table 8.5 The summary of existing (cross-sectional) studies examining orthorexia nervosa and mindfulness and/or mindful eating among adults

| Author(s) and year | Objective(s) of the study | Sample characteristics | Methods | Results | Conclusion |
|---|---|---|---|---|---|
| Strahler, 2021 | • To investigate the relationship between mindfulness and healthy orthorexia and orthorexia nervosa.<br>• H1: Healthy orthorexia is positively linked to mindfulness, while orthorexia nervosa shows the opposite pattern. | Germany: 389 adults (314 women)<br>$M_{age} = 27.17 \pm 10.64$ years<br>$M_{BMI} = 22.99 \pm 4.59$ kg/m$^2$ | • The Teruel Orthorexia Scale<br>• The Freiburg Mindfulness Inventory | • Healthy orthorexia was positively linked to mindfulness, while orthorexia nervosa was negatively associated with mindfulness.<br>• Mindfulness correlated with healthy orthorexia more strongly in women. | • Mindfulness encourages eating healthily and may protect against eating-related pathologies. |
| Kalika, Egan & Mantzios, 2022 | • To explore emotional eating, restrictive eating and external eating in a vegan population.<br>• To explore whether mindful eating and self-compassion have an impact on orthorexia nervosa. | United Kingdom; 313 adults following a vegan diet (287 women) aged 18 years or over<br>$M_{age} = 37.44 \pm 12.33$ years<br>$M_{BMI} = 24.86 \pm 4.87$ kg/m$^2$ | • The Düsseldorf Orthorexia Scale<br>• The Mindful Eating Behaviour Scale<br>• Sussex-Oxford Compassion Scales | • There was no relationship between orthorexia nervosa and mindful eating.<br>• High levels of orthorexia nervosa were associated with high levels of restrained eating and low levels of self-compassion. | • Self-compassion interventions could be a useful addition to support individuals who engage in restrictive eating and display orthorexic behaviours. |

Table 8.5 (cont.– Part A)

| Author(s) and year | Objective(s) of the study | Sample characteristics | Methods | Results | Conclusion |
|---|---|---|---|---|---|
| | • H1: Emotional eating and restrained eating are positively associated with orthorexia nervosa.<br>• H2: Self-compassion and potentially most aspects of mindful eating will be negatively correlated with orthorexia nervosa. | | • Salzburg Emotional Eating Scale<br>• Dutch Eating Behaviour Questionnaire | • Individuals with high levels of orthorexia nervosa displayed low levels of self-compassion and high levels of restrained eating.<br>• Self-compassion mediated the relationship between restrictive eating and orthorexia nervosa. | |
| Miley et al., 2022 | • To investigate the relationship between perfectionism, mindful eating and orthorexia nervosa. | United Kingdom; 670 adults (588 women) aged between 18 and 74 years<br>Median$_{age}$ = 39 years<br>$M_{BMI}$ = 28.19 ± 5.51 kg m$^2$ | • The Düsseldorf Orthorexia Scale<br>• The Mindful Eating Behaviour Scale<br>• The Big-Three Perfectionism Scale – Short Form | • Orthorexia nervosa was positively associated with perfectionism and focused eating (a facet of mindful eating).<br>• Orthorexia nervosa was negatively linked to 'eating with awareness' (a facet of mindful eating).<br>• Rigid perfectionism and focused eating demonstrated a predictive positive relationship with orthorexia nervosa. | • Mindful eating should be recognised by its different components (the findings confirm the complexity of mindful eating as a concept). |

**Table 8.5 (cont.– Part B)**

| Author(s) and year | Objective(s) of the study | Sample characteristics | Methods | Results | Conclusion |
|---|---|---|---|---|---|
| Demirer & Yardımcı, 2023 | • To investigate the relationship between mindful eating and orthorexia nervosa. | Turkey; 197 adults (105 women) aged between 19 and 64 years $M_{age} = 30.60 \pm 6.80$ years $M_{BMI} = 23.78 \pm 4.15$ kg/m$^2$ | • The ORTO–15 • The Mindful Eating Questionnaire • The SCOFF test • The Eating Attitudes Test–26 | • Orthorexia nervosa was negatively associated with mindful eating and abnormal eating behaviour. • Individuals with orthorexia nervosa demonstrated higher levels of emotional eating and conscious eating (facet of mindful eating) than those who do not have orthorexia nervosa. • Mindful eating and abnormal eating behaviour demonstrated a predictive negative relationship with orthorexia nervosa. | • Determination of the mindful eating status of individuals with orthorexia nervosa is of great importance to determine the criteria for diagnosis and treatment. |

**Table 8.5 (cont.– Part C)**

| Author(s) and year | Objective(s) of the study | Sample characteristics | Methods | Results | Conclusion |
|---|---|---|---|---|---|
| Kalika et al., 2023 | • To explore the association between orthorexia nervosa, mindfulness, mindful eating, self-compassion and eating-disordered quality of life in a female population.<br>• To explore whether mindful eating, self-compassion and mindfulness moderate the relationship between orthorexia nervosa and eating-disordered quality of life.<br>• H1: Mindful eating, mindfulness and self-compassion are negatively associated with orthorexia nervosa.<br>• H2: Women with high orthorexic tendencies demonstrate a lower quality of life. | United Kingdom; 288 women aged 18 years or over<br><br>$M_{age}$ =24.79±7.08 years<br>$M_{BMI}$ =24.26±6.45 kg/m$^2$ | • The Orthorexia Nervosa Inventory<br>• The Five-Facet Mindfulness Questionnaire – Short Form<br>• The Self-Compassion Scale – Short Form<br>• The Eating Disorder Quality of Life | • High levels of orthorexia nervosa were associated with low levels of focused eating, hunger and satiety, eating with awareness (facets of mindful eating), mindfulness and self-compassion.<br>• Women with high levels of orthorexia nervosa displayed lower levels of quality of life.<br>• Self-compassion and awareness (a facet of mindfulness) moderated the relationship between orthorexia nervosa and eating-disordered quality of life. | • Orthorexia nervosa was negatively associated with mindful eating, mindfulness and self-compassion. |

Table 8.5 (cont.– Part D)

| Author(s) and year | Objective(s) of the study | Sample characteristics | Methods | Results | Conclusion |
|---|---|---|---|---|---|
| Thorne, Hussain & Mantzios, 2023 | • To assess relationships between orthorexia nervosa, mindful eating, and feelings of guilt and shame. | United Kingdom; c176 undergraduate students (140 women) aged between 18 and 40 years $M_{age}$ = 21.7±1.9 years $M_{BMI}$ = 24.06±4.72 kg/m$^2$ | • Düsseldorf Orthorexia Scale <br> • The Mindful Eating Behaviour Scale <br> • The Weight- and Body-Related Shame and Guilt Scale | • Orthorexia nervosa was negatively associated with mindful eating, specifically, focused eating, hunger and satiety, and eating with awareness. <br> • Orthorexia nervosa was positively associated with guilt and shame. <br> • Guilt and shame mediated the relationship between orthorexia nervosa and mindful eating. | • Guilt and shame could explain the association between mindful eating and orthorexia nervosa. |

health-related beliefs and behaviours. Orthorexia nervosa would be associated with health locus of control, which concerns the belief that health is or is not in one's control (Nazareth et al., 2016). Little research has explored whether individuals with orthorexia nervosa believe that they have control over their health. It has been suggested that orthorexic symptomatology would be linked to a high internal and low external health locus of control (Oberle, Klare & Patyk, 2019). This would mean that individuals with orthorexia nervosa believe strongly that they can control their health condition and that their behaviours and actions determine health-related outcomes, and they tend to believe less that health outcomes are contingent on outside factors (e.g. doctors, other people, chance). Notwithstanding this, no statistical difference was found regarding the exhibition of a higher internal and lower external health locus of control between individuals presenting symptoms of orthorexia nervosa compared with the healthy eating group and the normal eating group (Oberle, Klare & Patyk, 2019). Up to now, only one cross-cultural study has examined whether the health behaviours, beliefs and symptoms are associated with orthorexia nervosa (Oberle, Klare & Patyk, 2019) and one mixed-methods study has investigated how conceptualisations of health and healthy eating are construed in the context of orthorexia nervosa (Greville-Harris et al., 2022) (Table 8.6).

Recent evidence suggests that orthorexia nervosa symptoms may stem, in part, from having a health-focused self-concept (i.e. overvaluing the importance of health for self-definition and self-worth) (Tabri, Yung & Elliott, 2022). Some qualitative literature indicates a link between beliefs about health control and orthorexia nervosa, suggesting that orthorexia nervosa might be associated with a perceived need for control of health (Cheshire, Berry & Fixsen, 2020) as well as perceived control of other areas of life felt uncontrollable (Greville-Harris et al., 2020). In addition, one exploratory qualitative research (Cheshire, Berry & Fixsen, 2020) found that individuals who self-identified as having orthorexia nervosa reported worries about health as a trigger for their symptoms.

### 8.4.1 Physical Activity

Orthorexia nervosa is not only positively linked to restriction on healthy eating (caring about following their schedules for meals, preoccupation with the amount of each nutrient included in the diet, eating special foods, and spending a considerable amount of time preparing their meals) but also to dissatisfaction with physical appearance (feeling concerned or dissatisfied with their physical appearance, concentrating on improving physical appearance while exercising), as well as to frequent exercising (following strict schedules for exercise, feeling guilty about not being able to exercise as often as wanted) in

Table 8.6 The summary of existing studies evaluating health beliefs and health behaviours linked to orthorexia nervosa

| Author(s) and year | Objective(s) of the study | Sample characteristics | Methods | Results | Conclusion |
|---|---|---|---|---|---|
| Greville-Harris et al., 2022 | • To investigate how individuals at risk for orthorexia nervosa conceptualise health and healthy eating.<br>• To examine whether health anxiety and beliefs in health controllability are relevant factors in the psychopathology of orthorexia nervosa. | United Kingdom; the quantitative section of the study: 362 adults (204 women) aged 18 years and over<br><br>$M_{age} = 27.79 \pm 8.89$ years<br><br>$M_{BMI} = 24.73 \pm 5.26$ kg/m$^2$<br><br>The qualitative section of the study: 141 adults being at risk of orthorexia nervosa (94 women)<br><br>$M_{age} = 28.51 \pm 8.22$ years<br><br>$M_{BMI} = 24.82 \pm 5.34$ kg/m$^2$ | • The Düsseldorf Orthorexia Scale<br>• The Eating Habits Questionnaire<br>• The Health Anxiety Questionnaire<br>• The Multidimensional Health Locus of Control Scale (Form A): Internality Subscale | • Four themes were generated from the qualitative data: 'health is more than thin ideals'; 'healthy food equals a healthy mind'; 'a body that works for you' and 'taking control of your body'.<br>• The quantitative analysis revealed that higher levels of health anxiety and beliefs in health controllability predicted symptomatology of orthorexia nervosa | • Both qualitative and quantitative data suggest that beliefs and emotions around health and healthy eating are fundamental to orthorexia nervosa.<br>• Both health anxiety and health controllability are important targets for future investigation. |

**Table 8.6 (cont.)**

| Author(s) and year | Objective(s) of the study | Sample characteristics | Methods | Results | Conclusion |
|---|---|---|---|---|---|
| Oberle, Klare & Patyk, 2019 | • To evaluate the health behaviours, beliefs and symptoms associated with orthorexia nervosa. <br><br> H1: The group presenting symptoms of orthorexia nervosa would report greater use of nutritional supplements and complementary and alternative medicine techniques and would endorse more reasons for doing so to improve both physical and psychological health in comparison to two control groups, including a normal eating control group and a healthy eating control group. | United States; 180 students (150 women) aged 18 to 48 years. <br><br> $M_{age} = 21.43 \pm 3.55$ years. <br><br> Group presenting symptoms of orthorexia nervosa: $n = 47$ <br><br> Normal eating control group: $n = 50$ <br><br> Healthy eating control group: $n = 83$ | • The Eating Habits Questionnaire <br> • The Supplements and Complementary and Alternative Medicine Questionnaire <br> • The Multidimensional Health Locus of Control Questionnaire <br> • The Cohen-Hoberman Inventory of Physical Symptoms | • H1 was partially supported: The group presenting symptoms of orthorexia nervosa reported greater use of both supplements and alternative medicine techniques (most notably, B vitamins, fish oil, protein powders and yoga) when compared to the normal eating group; however, these health behaviours did not significantly differ between the group presenting symptoms of orthorexia nervosa. | • The present study was the first to empirically demonstrate that orthorexic symptoms are associated not only with increased intake of nutritional supplements and increased participation in complementary and alternative medicine techniques, but also with poorer physical health, which is contrary to their goal of achieving perfect health. |

**Table 8.6 (cont.)**

| Author(s) and year | Objective(s) of the study | Sample characteristics | Methods | Results | Conclusion |
|---|---|---|---|---|---|
| | H2: The group presenting symptoms of orthorexia nervosa would exhibit a higher internal and lower external health locus of control in comparison to the normal eating control group. | | | and the healthy eating control group • H2 and H3 were not supported: none of the groups differed on internal or external health locus of control. • H4 was supported. | • Contrary to the goal of achieving perfect health, individuals presenting symptoms of orthorexia nervosa experience diminished physical health. |
| | H3: The group presenting symptoms of orthorexia nervosa would exhibit a lower internal and higher external health locus of control in comparison to both control groups. | | | | |
| | H4: The group presenting symptoms of orthorexia nervosa would complain of more symptoms associated with poor physical health in comparison to both control groups. | | | | |

adult gym members (Almeida, Vieira Borba & Santos, 2018). It was found that 61% of individuals with orthorexia nervosa 'always' exercised more than three times per week (Almeida, Vieira Borba & Santos, 2018). More frequent exercising was associated with orthorexia nervosa in women (Aksoydan & Camci, 2009). Female athletes (who were involved in competitive or vigorous fitness programmes and participated in no less than three 1.5-hour exercise sessions per week for at least three years) had significantly higher levels of orthorexia nervosa symptomatology compared to their sedentary counterparts (Segura-García et al., 2012). Individuals engaging in more sports activity had a higher orthorexia nervosa symptom severity compared to those who did not engage in any sport (Foyster et al., 2023; Varga et al., 2014). More precisely, athletes performing sports for more than 150 minutes/week and those practising sports for less than 150 minutes/week had significantly higher levels of orthorexia nervosa symptomatology in comparison with inactive individuals (Bert et al., 2019). Furthermore, practising endurance sports for more than 150 minutes/week was linked with higher levels of orthorexia nervosa (Bert et al., 2019). Individuals with a high risk of orthorexia nervosa spent the most amount of time training, they felt guiltier if they skipped a training, and they paid more attention to the amount of calories they burnt during training in comparison with those with moderate and low risk of orthorexia nervosa (Kiss-Leizer, Tóth-Király & Rigó, 2019). Orthorexia nervosa symptomatology was related to higher exercise activity levels, namely, more time spent on strength training and aerobic exercises in university students (Oberle, Watkins & Burkot, 2018). Moreover, it was associated with relatively greater strength-training exercises in male than in female students (Oberle, Watkins & Burkot, 2018). Orthorexia nervosa was associated with higher levels of health anxiety (independently from the actual physical condition), the motivation for healthy behaviours (in the context of mood modification, weight control, social desirability and healthy lifestyle) and 'unhealthy' sports habits (the hours spent on sports activities on an average week, feeling guilty if skipping training, monitoring of calorie burnt during training and the frequency of weekly occasions of doing sport) in the general population (Kiss-Leizer, Tóth-Király & Rigó, 2019).

Orthorexia nervosa symptomatology was linked to different exercise motivations, namely internal motivation to exercise (i.e. exercising due to internal pressures to exercise and guilt over missed sessions, due to the value of the benefits of exercise, due to natural enjoyment of exercise activities), psychological improvement motivations, social improvement motivations, health improvement motivations and body improvement motivations in undergraduate students (Oberle, Watkins & Burkot, 2018). More precisely, orthorexia nervosa symptomatology was related to higher levels of motivation for improvements in physical health (i.e. exercising to achieve positive health and avoid ill health), in fitness that is relevant to physical health (i.e. exercising to achieve strength, endurance, nimbleness and low body fat), in psychological health (i.e. exercising for stress management, revitalisation, enjoyment and challenge) and in social relationships (i.e. exercising to spend time with others, compete and be recognised for accomplishments with exercise). Other motives, such as mood modification (i.e. monitoring health in a negative affective state), weight control (i.e. being healthy to achieve desired weight), social desirability (i.e. being healthy to gain social support) and healthy lifestyle (i.e. being healthy has positive consequences) were related to orthorexia nervosa in the general population (Kiss-Leizer, Tóth-Király & Rigó, 2019). Orthorexia nervosa was also found to be negatively related to adaptive eating motivations, including 'hunger' and 'pleasure' (indicating that these motives do not drive individuals with orthorexia for food choices and that their eating behaviours may be less intuitive), and positively linked to eating motivations considered to be core components of orthorexia nervosa, such as 'health', 'natural concern' and 'social image' (Foyster et al., 2023). In addition, orthorexia nervosa was also associated with 'weight control', indicating that a desire to manipulate weight and shape may be a strong motivator for food choices in individuals with orthorexia nervosa (Foyster et al., 2023).

Orthorexia nervosa symptomatology was linked to higher levels of exercise addiction in fitness centre members (Rudolph, 2018), university students (Oberle, Watkins & Burkot, 2018) and male college students (White, Berry & Rodgers, 2020). In women, both orthorexia nervosa and exercise addiction were positively related to anxiety (with a stronger correlation for orthorexia nervosa). While in men, both behaviours were associated with the personality trait conscientiousness (to a similar extent) (Strahler et al., 2021). A previous meta-analysis on the association of orthorexia nervosa with exercise measures and exercise addiction, including 10,134 individuals (Strahler, Wachten & Mueller-Alcazar, 2021), demonstrated weak and moderate relationships with general exercise and exercise addiction respectively, and comparable relationships between orthorexia nervosa and exercise in women and men. One study established that orthorexia nervosa was not related to addiction to exercise among exercise practitioners (Freire et al., 2020).

To sum up, individuals with orthorexia nervosa are internally driven to engage in physical activity as these strong motivations lead to exercise addiction and a compulsive need to follow a rigid schedule of intensive exercise (Oberle, Watkins & Burkot, 2018). It has been theorised that individuals with orthorexia nervosa might not get pleasure from exercising (Kiss-Leizer, Tóth-Király & Rigó, 2019), and they might treat physical activity as a method for 'effective' emotional and behavioural self-regulation. Like healthy eating, they might also be preoccupied with excessive exercise (Kiss-Leizer, Tóth-Király & Rigó, 2019). Compulsive or excessive exercise has been linked to orthorexia nervosa symptomatology in previous studies (Foyster et al., 2023; Håman, Lindgren & Prell, 2017; Oberle, Watkins & Burkot, 2018; Rudolph, 2018) suggesting that the addition of this behaviour to the diagnostic criteria or assessment for orthorexia nervosa may capture the phenomenon more comprehensively. However, it is important to note that although excessive exercise is likewise characteristic of patients with eating disorders, it is not considered a diagnostic criterion in anorexia nervosa despite significant co-occurrence (Sanzari & Hormes, 2023). In line with eating disorders, it is possible that physical activity, due to its unique characteristics (i.e. excessive exercise), might be considered a symptom of orthorexia nervosa, with the same underlying pathological background as the unhealthy way of healthy eating (Kiss-Leizer, Tóth-Király & Rigó, 2019). Therefore, additional criteria specifically intended to distinguish orthorexia nervosa from other related disorders would be beneficial for the measurement of this phenomenon and should be part of the diagnostic criteria for orthorexia nervosa (e.g. exercise-related symptoms, body shape/weight concerns, fear of eating certain foods; Sanzari & Hormes, 2023). Excessive physical activity might be considered an important potential predictor factor of orthorexia nervosa. Nonetheless, more research is needed to support this assumption.

## 8.5 Body Image

To what extent is body image related to orthorexia nervosa? A growing number of studies address this question. However, findings vary depending on the context and do not provide evidence as to whether or not body image disturbance (Pauzé et al., 2021) should be considered a diagnostic feature of orthorexia nervosa. There is evidence to suppose that body image concerns may play a part in orthorexia nervosa and those which do not support the previous findings. The findings have revealed that individuals with orthorexia nervosa experience high levels of body dissatisfaction (e.g. Barnes & Caltabiano, 2017; Barthels, Kisser & Pietrowsky, 2021; Haddad et al., 2019) and body weight and shape concerns (Bartel et al., 2020; Levin et al., 2023). Overweight preoccupation, appearance orientation and the presence of an eating disorder history were found to be significant predictors of orthorexia nervosa in adults (Barnes & Caltabiano, 2017). In yoga practitioners, orthorexia nervosa was predicted, among others, by higher levels of drive for thinness and dysfunctional beliefs about appearance (Domingues & Carmo, 2021). It was identified that orthorexia nervosa was linked to an unhealthy body-self relationship among women (Brytek-Matera et al., 2016). Women with orthorexia nervosa were more likely to continually include exercise activities into their lifestyle (fitness orientation), focus on dieting, eating restraint and weight vigilance (overweight preoccupation), take notice of their appearance (appearance orientation) and lead a physically healthy lifestyle (health orientation). In addition, they were less likely to be satisfied with discrete parts of their appearance (Brytek-Matera et al., 2016). Female fitness centre participants who exercised more frequently were more willing to both agree with and adopt and/or accept the Western social ideal of slimness, as well as exhibiting a greater level of anxiety with their bodies (social physique anxiety) and had higher levels of symptoms of orthorexia nervosa, whereas in male fitness centre participants, the adaptation and/or acceptance of Western social ideals of muscularity was related to orthorexia nervosa symptomatology (Eriksson et al., 2008). Men with higher levels of internalisation of the ideal muscular body (Aksoydan & Camci, 2009), male college students with higher levels of muscularity-oriented behaviours, thin-ideal internalisation and athletic-ideal internalisation (White, Berry & Rodgers, 2020) and individuals who perceived themselves as having a relatively muscular, lean body type (Oberle & Lipschuetz, 2018) presented high levels of orthorexia nervosa symptomatology. It has been revealed that predictors of orthorexia nervosa depend on sex in the general population (Stutts, 2020). Weight/shape concerns, weight-related routine restraint, stress and negative emotions predicted orthorexia nervosa in women. Overvaluation of weight and shape was found to be the only component of body image (besides overvaluation, dissatisfaction, preoccupation, body checking and body image avoidance) to predict orthorexia nervosa in adult women uniquely (Messer et al., 2022). In comparison, weight-related routine restraint, emotional eating, stress and well-being were found to be significant predictors of orthorexia nervosa in men (Stutts, 2020).

Orthorexic behaviours and social anxiety symptoms predicted the symptomatology of muscle dysmorphia (the preoccupation with the idea that one's body is not sufficiently lean and muscular) in bodybuilders (Cerea et al., 2018). Also, in university students, high levels of desire for size, appearance anxiety/avoidance and functional impairment (diagnostic factors associated with muscle dysmorphia) were related to orthorexia nervosa (Gorrasi et al., 2020). Thus, the dysfunctional eating patterns characterised by a rigid, healthy diet might trigger engagement in muscle dysmorphia symptoms and behaviours (Cerea et al., 2018). High levels of orthorexic eating behaviour were found to mediate the association between high levels of perfectionism and muscle dysmorphic disorder in young male adults (Merhy et al., 2023). In individuals with orthorexia nervosa, weight control had priority over health as the primary motive for food choice and selection (Bartel et al., 2020; Depa et al., 2019). These findings suggest that some individuals with orthorexia nervosa might not be exclusively concerned about health but also body image or body weight.

On the other hand, no links were found between orthorexia nervosa and upward physical appearance comparison in female and male adults (Scheiber, Diehl & Karmasin, 2023), body dissatisfaction in female and male adults (Freire et al., 2020; Scheiber, Diehl & Karmasin, 2023; Yakın, Raynal & Chabrol, 2022) or solely in men (Zakhour et al., 2021), body satisfaction with the lower body (i.e. waist/midsection, abdomen, hips, thighs, legs) and weight in female and male adults (Plichta, Jeżewska-Zychowicz & Gębski, 2019), and body uneasiness solely in male adults (Brytek-Matera et al., 2017).

Despite the contradictory findings, orthorexia nervosa seems to be associated with specific body image attitudes. It should be pointed out that all described studies relied on self-report measures, and no objective body measures were included (Pauzé et al., 2021). Therefore, a previous study (Pauzé et al., 2021) investigated the existence of a potential link between orthorexia nervosa symptomatology and body image distortion in a non-clinical sample, with both explicit and implicit measures. The findings revealed that orthorexia nervosa was positively associated with implicit body image attitudes, namely body fat dissatisfaction and muscularity dissatisfaction, meaning that individuals with orthorexia nervosa had the desire to have less body fat in their overall body, chest or breast area, abdomen area, hips area and be more muscular on the chest or breast. Orthorexia nervosa was also positively related to explicit body image attitudes, namely investment in physical health and leading a healthy lifestyle, appearance and physical fitness, as well as overweight preoccupation. Orthorexia nervosa was not linked to implicit body fat distortion as well as explicit body size distortion. However, orthorexia nervosa was associated with implicit abdomen muscularity distortion, which means that individuals with orthorexia under-estimated their abdominal muscularity. Finally, orthorexia nervosa symptomatology was predicted mainly by explicit overweight preoccupation, explicit investment in physical health and leading a healthy lifestyle and implicit muscularity distortion. These findings suggest that orthorexia nervosa symptomatology is positively associated with body image attitudes and distortion in a non-clinical sample. It has also been suggested that individuals with orthorexia nervosa may exhibit a 'healthy ideal body image' through the value of and investment in physical health, fitness and weight control (Pauzé et al., 2021).

## 8.6 Emotion Regulation

Emotion regulation refers to the processes involved in shaping which emotions one experiences, when emotions are experienced, and how these emotions are experienced and expressed (Gross, 1998). Emotion regulation pertains to monitoring, identifying, evaluating, experiencing, expressing and modifying emotions in terms of intensity, form and duration of feelings, emotion-related physiological states and behaviours (Kok, 2020). According to Gratz and Roemer (2004), the authors of the Difficulties in Emotion Regulation Scale, emotion regulation may be conceptualised as involving the (1) awareness and understanding of emotions, (2) acceptance of emotions, (3) ability to control impulsive behaviours and behave by desired goals when experiencing negative emotions, and (4) ability to use situationally appropriate emotion regulation strategies flexibly to modulate emotional responses as desired to meet individual goals and situational demands. The relative absence of any or all of these abilities would indicate the presence of difficulties in emotion regulation or emotion dysregulation. Adaptive emotion regulation strategies involve modulating the experience of intensive emotions to facilitate achieving desired goals rather than eliminating certain emotions (Gratz & Roemer, 2004). Today, there are only three studies (Obeid et al., 2021; Vuillier et al., 2020; Strahler et al., 2022) to assess emotion regulation in orthorexia nervosa. In these three studies, the researchers used the Difficulties in Emotion Regulation Scale (Table 8.7).

We can assume that orthorexic eating may be a form of emotion regulation used when other strategies are not useful or fail or may be rooted in beliefs about a lack of capacity to use emotion regulation strategies when needed (Strahler et al., 2022). Orthorexic eating is then used to gain feelings of security by focusing on healthy eating. We can also suppose that restrictive dietary rules around healthy eating could be considered a coping strategy to feel 'perfect' and in control (Greville-Harris, Smithson & Karl, 2020). Thus, dietary rules can increase levels of perceived control to better cope with difficult emotions. This may be predominantly the situation if the individuals do not acknowledge their emotional responses and consider the absence of other approaches to make them feel better. According to the author of this book, it is worth considering whether individuals with orthorexia nervosa, instead of focusing on their emotions and emotional responses, turn their attention to their tasks (e.g. being in good health). However, they may be unable to deal with their difficult emotions, resulting in a reluctance to confront their emotions and their regulation. It may seem that individuals with orthorexia nervosa try to temporarily avoid negative emotions because they have limited access to adaptive emotion regulation strategies. In orthorexia nervosa, a self-imposed dietary restriction may presumably serve as an alternative, maladaptive strategy of emotion regulation. The previous study (Pauligk et al., 2021) suggests that over-control in patients with anorexia nervosa may have negative affective consequences on a short (minutes) as well as a longer timescale (days). It could be the same in the case of individuals with orthorexia nervosa, but it has to be empirically proved.

Table 8.7 The summary of existing (cross-sectional) studies examining the relationship between orthorexia nervosa and emotion regulation among adults

| Author(s) and year | Objective(s) of the study | Sample characteristics | Methods | Results | Conclusion |
|---|---|---|---|---|---|
| Vuillier, Robertson & Greville-Harris, 2020 | • To assess emotion regulation difficulties and alexithymia in a sample of individuals with orthorexia tendencies.<br><br>H1: Orthorexic tendencies would be positively associated with alexithymia and emotion regulation difficulties. | Convenience sampling; United Kingdom; 196 adults (167 women) aged 18–66 years<br><br>$M_{age}$ = 27.90 ± 12.90 years<br><br>$M_{BMI}$ = 22.89 ± 3.64 kg/m$^2$ | • The ORTO-15 (reduced to ORTO-7CS – corrected scoring)<br>• The Difficulties in Emotion Regulation Scale (DERS–16)<br>• The Toronto Alexithymia Scale<br>• The Eating Attitudes Test | • Difficulties regulating emotions and identifying feelings were associated with symptoms of orthorexia nervosa.<br>• Individuals with high orthorexic tendencies had more difficulties identifying and accepting their feelings, resisting impulses, engaging in goal-directed behaviours and finding the right strategies when upset compared to people with low orthorexic tendencies. | • Individuals with orthorexic tendencies may share similar difficulties identifying and regulating their emotions to other eating diagnosable disorders.<br>• Symptoms of orthorexia nervosa were not associated with difficulties describing emotions, unlike other eating disorders.<br>• Orthorexic behaviour may be used as a coping strategy to feel in control in those participants who have poor emotion regulation abilities. |

**Table 8.7 (cont.)**

| Author(s) and year | Objective(s) of the study | Sample characteristics | Methods | Results | Conclusion |
|---|---|---|---|---|---|
| Obeid et al., 2021 | • To investigate the association between orthorexia nervosa and difficulties identifying, describing and regulating emotions.<br><br>H1: Emotion regulation difficulties and alexithymia would be linked to higher levels of orthorexia nervosa. | Snowball sampling<br><br>Lebanon;<br>787 adults (532 women)<br><br>$M_{age} = 26.33 \pm 12.16$ years<br><br>$M_{BMI} = 24.06 \pm 4.72 \, kg/m^2$ | • The ORTO-R<br>• The Difficulty in Emotion Regulation Scale (DERS–16)<br>• The Toronto Alexithymia Scale<br>• The Eating Attitudes Test | • Orthorexia nervosa was associated with higher levels of alexithymia, difficulties in emotion regulation, physical activity and disordered eating attitudes.<br>• Higher levels of emotion dysregulation, lower levels of alexithymia and more disordered eating attitudes predicted higher levels of orthorexia nervosa. | • Difficulties identifying, describing and regulating one's own emotions may be a risk factor for orthorexia nervosa. |

Table 8.7 (cont.)

| Author(s) and year | Objective(s) of the study | Sample characteristics | Methods | Results | Conclusion |
|---|---|---|---|---|---|
| Strahler et al., 2022 | • To investigate the associations of emotion regulation difficulties and insecure attachment styles with orthorexia nervosa and healthy orthorexia . <br><br> • To explore the mediating role of difficulties in emotion regulation for the association between insecure attachment and orthorexia nervosa. | Convenience sampling; Germany; 399 adults (266 women) aged between 16 and 82 years <br><br> $M_{age} = 30.53 \pm 12.90$ years <br><br> $M_{BMI} = 22.89 \pm 3.64\,kg/m^2$ | • The Teruel Orthorexia Scale <br><br> • The Difficulties in Emotion Regulation Scale (DERS–36) <br><br> • The Experiences in Close Relationships – Revised Questionnaire <br><br> • The Depression-Anxiety-Stress Scales | • Orthorexia nervosa was positively associated with difficulties in emotion regulation, attachment-related anxiety and avoidance. <br><br> • Healthy orthorexia was only negatively linked to a lack of emotional awareness. <br><br> • Non-acceptance of emotional responses and impulse control difficulties fully mediated the relationship between attachment style and orthorexia nervosa. In addition, affective symptoms partially moderated this association. | • Individuals with higher orthorexia nervosa tendencies demonstrated increased difficulties in emotion regulation and a more insecure attachment pattern. <br><br> • Difficulties in emotion regulation and insecure attachment style should be considered as potential vulnerability factors or diagnostic criteria for orthorexia nervosa. |

The author of this book goes along with Pauligk and colleagues' (2021) view that while over-controlled behaviour may be experienced as a helpful way to reduce tension in the short term, it may increase tension in the long run. In other words, self-imposed food rules can temporarily reduce the intensity of emotions but deteriorate the ability to deal with emotions in the long term. This statement requires empirical and clinical evidence among individuals with orthorexia nervosa. A future study should provide evidence of whether difficulties in emotion regulation are one of the social-emotional factors contributing to the development and maintenance of orthorexia nervosa, as with eating disorders (Leppanen et al., 2022).

# 9 Nutritional Characteristics of Orthorexia Nervosa

## 9.1 Dietary Patterns

Several dietary patterns (e.g. the 'prudent diet' being high in fruit and vegetables, legumes, fish and whole grains, the 'Western diet' being higher in processed meats, red meats, French fries, sweets and desserts and refined grains) have been identified and described in the scientific literature up to now (Green, 2015). Previous research has established that individuals with orthorexia nervosa are less likely to consume saturated fats or animal fat products (Grammatikopoulou et al., 2018), products high in sugar, snacks, dressings and refined bread (Plichta & Jeżewska-Zychowicz, 2019; Plichta, Jeżewska-Zychowicz & Gębski, 2019). Daily bread consumption amount and carbohydrate intake in individuals with orthorexia nervosa were found to be significantly lower than in those without orthorexia nervosa (Yassıbaş & Gençer Bingöl, 2023). Moreover, the percentage of individuals who do not consume bread was approximately three times higher among individuals with orthorexia nervosa compared to those without orthorexia nervosa. In contrast, individuals with orthorexia nervosa are more likely to consume vegetables, fruits, nuts, legumes, seeds and meat (Plichta & Jeżewska-Zychowicz, 2019; Plichta, Jeżewska-Zychowicz & Gębski, 2019). Regarding the daily energy and nutrient intake in individuals with orthorexia nervosa, carbohydrate, soluble fibre and insoluble fibre intake was significantly lower. In contrast, the intake of protein and fat percentages (according to energy) were significantly higher in comparison with individuals without orthorexia nervosa (Yassıbaş & Gençer Bingöl, 2023). Consumption of protein, carbohydrate, fat, monounsaturated fat, polyunsaturated fat, fibre and salt (Grammatikopoulou et al., 2018) and taking dietary supplements (Almeida, Vieira Borba & Santos, 2018) were found to be unrelated to orthorexia nervosa.

It has been demonstrated that individuals with orthorexia nervosa less frequently consume sugar-rich and refined products, and their diet contains less sugar and salt in comparison with those with eating disorders and healthy ones (Plichta & Jeżewska-Zychowicz, 2019). Moreover, a higher percentage of them had four or more meals daily, consumed regular meals, had a gap of three to four hours between meals, and did not skip midday meals and dinner. Also, those who engaged in alternative food networks, characterised by buying organic, locally grown, sustainably grown, artisanal foods (Barnett et al., 2016), and those who more frequently shopped in health food stores (Varga et al., 2014) were more likely to have orthorexia nervosa (Barnett et al., 2016), similar to those who substituted lunch or dinner with fruit or salads (Bagci Bosi et al., 2007).

Previous research findings into food intolerance have been contradictory. On the one hand, having two or more food intolerances makes individuals more likely to have orthorexia nervosa (Missbach et al., 2015). On the other hand, in other studies, having a food intolerance or avoiding certain foods due to a food allergy or being medically prescribed was unrelated to orthorexia nervosa (Barnes & Caltabiano, 2017; Reynolds, 2018). Individuals with allergies and intolerances did not display higher levels of orthorexic eating behaviour than those without allergies and intolerances (Barthels, Bamberg & Pietrowsky, 2022). However, in this group, orthorexic eating behaviour was positively associated with the number of allergy-related consequences (such as only eating self-prepared food, checking ingredients and avoiding social events) and the perceived severity of the allergic symptoms (Barthels, Bamberg & Pietrowsky, 2022).

Studying dietary patterns can guide nutrition intervention and education (Hu, 2002) in individuals with orthorexia nervosa. In contrast to the traditional analytical approach used in nutritional epidemiology, dietary pattern analysis considers the overall diet rather than individual nutrients or foods (Hu, 2002). There are three statistical methods for defining dietary patterns (they cannot be measured directly): factor analysis, cluster analysis and dietary indices. Factor analysis uses information reported on food frequency questionnaires or in dietary records to identify common underlying factors or patterns of food consumption. In contrast to factor analysis, cluster analysis aggregates individuals into relatively homogeneous subgroups (clusters) with similar diets. Dietary indices (e.g. the healthy eating index, the diet quality index and the dietary diversity score) assess overall diet quality. These indices are typically based on dietary recommendations (Hu, 2002). Research to evaluate the validity of dietary patterns and whether they predict 'disease' risk in individuals with orthorexia nervosa would be beneficial.

## 9.2 Expert Commentary: Thoughts on Orthorexia Nervosa and Dieting Trends

by Professor Marle Alvarenga

**Marle Alvarenga**, PhD is external adviser in the Post-Graduation Program in Public Health Nutrition at University of São Paulo, Brazil, head of Specialized Group in Eating Disorders, Nutrition and Obesity (GENTA) and of the

Behavioral Nutrition Institute, both in São Paulo, Brazil. Her major research interests are eating behaviour and eating disorders. She has more than 90 published articles and 5 books on topics of interest. She is a speaker at conferences in Brazil and internationally, frequently lecturing about eating behaviour and eating disorders throughout Brazil and constantly being interviewed by the media.

Affiliation: Postgraduate Program in Nutrition in Public Health, School of Public Health, University of São Paulo, São Paulo, Brazil.

I got interested in orthorexia (ON) because of my work with eating disorders (ED). We published the first article that discussed this behaviour in Brazil (Martins et al., 2011) with a review of what had been published so far. After 12 years, the number of studies on ON is growing, and a discussion persists about whether or not it is an ED or even a new psychiatric disorder. Several scholars have written papers on the subject. As a dietitian, I focus on the importance of the ON concept to discuss healthy eating (Martins et al., 2011).

In the area of health and food, it is amazing how the fads and mismatched, fallacious, unscientific, and disordered discourses persist. What is healthy eating? Unfortunately, the widespread concept changes 'with the times', from vilifying to deifying a certain food or nutrient, or food 'practice' or diet.

The very term 'diet' is an example of inappropriate food intake and distortion. From its origin in dietetics, the medical knowledge that started caring for sick people's food in hospitals, and from its Greek origin diaita, meaning way of life, diet has become a restriction. Even dictionaries describe it as a 'medical prescription to a sick person or therapeutic deprivation of all or some foods'. Thus, diet became related essentially to slimming (often disguised as 'health').

In addition, even among health professionals, the focus of discussion on 'healthy eating' is usually only strictly biological, and adequate food is thought of as a diet that meets the nutritional recommendations. In fact, this definition depends on many factors, such as individual and family history, culture, religion, socio-economic aspects, personal experience, preferences and aversions, knowledge and beliefs, among others (Martins et al., 2011). Suppose this narrow idea about healthy eating and its erroneous association with 'diet' are present in today's cultures. How could they not impact the general public and even more so the people in the disordered eating spectrum?

In clinical care of ED, it has already been brought to our attention that the discourse of patients with anorexia nervosa has been changing – it is no longer focused on calories and diet/light foods but with a concern for fibre, vitamins, 'toxin', purity, being 'good for health', etc. The classic question 'how it all started' is no longer answered with 'a diet', but 'it all started when I decided to be healthier'!

A recent publication argues that ON 'is not a new psychiatric disorder but rather a new cultural manifestation of anorexia nervosa' (Bhattacharya et al., 2022). The authors also discuss the culture of dieting, which has only become worse, bringing up the fact that it has become almost an obligation due to the high preoccupation with achieving personal health as the principal defining factor of well-being (Crawford, 1980). As health thought frequently obtained via lifestyle modifications has become something persecutory – that judges and blames individuals for not fulfilling their 'social obligation' to be healthy – it brings up the issue of the moralisation of food related to ON (Bhattacharya et al., 2022).

This discussion about diet culture is complex; it changes focus but continues to affect thousands of people and make much money – despite its disastrous consequences for psychosocial health and the fact that it does not solve the obesity problem. It involves psychological, socio-anthropological and economic issues and is constructed and fed by various actors. However, how do we health professionals, especially those dealing with food and nutrition, contribute to this phenomenon?

As I started studying ON behaviour, I came across some specific evaluations, and these papers are growing – we have so far 5 studies that evaluated dietitians and 16 studies with nutrition students (e.g. Agopyan et al., 2019; Busatta et al., 2022; Tremelling et al., 2017; Villa et al., 2022).

We still have the problem of evaluating behaviour with no diagnostic criteria, done with several instruments (and today, a robust discussion about the inadequacy of some questionnaires, such as the ORTO-15 which is still the most used). In addition, the studies with the public do not provide a comparison with other professions or students in general, and there is no control group. In any case, the scores on the instruments assessing the frequency of so-called orthorexic behaviour are high in this audience.

Nevertheless, such studies raise some questions about the dietitian's vision of healthy eating. Would an orthorexic view result from excessive academic training and background and/or even be exclusively based on the nutritional quality of the diet?

It was argued that health professionals could be 'more prone' to ON behaviours due to their routine work addressing health and nutrition (Alvarenga et al., 2012).

A parallel with ED could be made. It is known that some studies find more risk behaviour for ED among nutrition students than among other careers. However, Reinstein et al. (1992) found that junior and senior students had better eating habits than freshmen. We can infer or believe that the course is not 'pathological' and does not teach ED behaviours, or orthorexic behaviours.

However, it is discussed that many people seek a course in nutrition because of excessive personal problems and concerns with the body and food. This question is even more relevant in times of social media and personalities who are an 'inspiration', even believing that dietitians do work similar to that of fit celebrities!

The name orthorexia refers to pathology and the neologism was created for this purpose. However, many nutritionists and lay people do not see a problem in the concept of clean eating, which is closely related to ON. This term is still little studied (Barrada & Roncero, 2018), but it is discussed that the adoption of 'clean eating' also incorporates strict gluten-free, dairy-free, sugar-free, grain-free, plant-based diets, or a combination thereof. The movement has been perpetuated by numerous unqualified health bloggers and celebrities and makes a connection with ON and even ARFID (avoidant/restrictive food intake disorder).

Bratman (the 'father' of ON) states that alternative diets can be safely followed, and that the development of ON would be a separate state. Also that the interest in healthy eating does not become pathological until there is a 'progression, a second stage of obsessive thinking, compulsive behaviour, self-punishment, escalating restriction, and other dynamics conventional to ED' (Reinstein et al., 1992). He states that in general the more complex the theory adopted by the individual with regard to the alternative diet, the more material it gives to the acceleration of the ON.

Bratman points out that most diet theories are clearly unscientific, pseudo-scientific or anti-scientific, as well as bizarre, but that following the rituals of these theories is the result of adherence to them rather than the expression of a pathology (Staudacher & Harer, 2018). Nevertheless, what if these restricted diets and this mistaken view of healthy eating is perpetuated by dietitians? Are we not the experts by training in food and nutrition? Celebrities can be great influencers, but the word of experts has much more truth.

The training and attitudes of nutritionists have been the focus of some of our work, showing stigma towards obesity – among professionals and students (Bratman, 1997; Cori, Petty & Alvarenga, 2015; Obara, Vivolo & Alvarenga, 2018; Alvarenga, et al., 2022) – and a restricted view of healthy eating, focusing only on the biological (Koritar & Alvarenga, 2017).

Our evaluation of ON among Brazilian dietitians, concluded (as others) that the ORTO-15 had poor psychometric properties. In any case, the responses revealed ON tendencies at a higher frequency than other studies with nutritionists to date (Alvarenga et al., 2012). The most prominent responses were for making food choices conditioned by worry about health status, evaluating food rather from nutritional quality than taste, believing that consuming healthy food may improve appearance, discrediting the influence of mood on eating behaviour and banning food choices considered as eating transgressions.

Results brought into the discussion again show the importance of deeply discussing healthy eating from a biopsychosocio-cultural point of view among professionals working with nutrition. How are we training these professionals, and what concept of healthy eating do they have (and probably disseminate)?

Today we have instruments with better psychometric quality (da Silva et al., 2021), which we used in a study in Brazil to evaluate ON among dietitians, gastrologists (who also have a background in food, but with a focus on cooking, culture and gastronomy) and a group with other professions. Using the Teruel Orthorexic Scale, we found that the dietitians scored lower for ON, and higher for what this instrument calls 'healthy orthorexia' (da Silva et al., 2021). This name is in itself very problematic and evaluated by questions such as 'I would rather eat a healthy food that is not very tasty than a tasty food that is not healthy' and 'I would rather eat little, but in a healthy way, than be satiated with a food that may not be healthy', which we see as equally 'problematic' behaviours with food. The path analysis used in this study did not point to profession as explaining the variance for ON scores, but rather age, body shape, concern about vegetarianism practice and risk behaviour for eating disorders (Takeda, 2022).

Nevertheless, we urgently need to 'take advantage' of the emergence of the concept of ON to discuss the fads in food, that is, the diets, and how the dietitians themselves are advertising and orientating healthy eating. Unfortunately, we have several reports of professionals who promote 'clean eating' and orthorexic ideas, advertising their diets and their ideas for their patients. It is not possible to believe that a person with problems with food and weight can adequately guide others, and for this reason, evaluating dietitians is important, but it is also necessary to think of a more holistic and critical formation since graduation, besides ethical and orientative guidelines from class entities seeking access to this problematic issue.

We certainly have a lot of research to do to better understand ON as a dysfunctional behaviour. In any case, Bratman's call to avoid pathologising alternative diets makes some sense, because people tend to believe what they read, the experts they trust, the communities they belong to, the media they follow, and are products of their culture. However, we must call attention to the damage of restrictive diets and educate people about their ineffectiveness and risks; and dietitians cannot be disseminators or facilitators of this kind of *upsetting* eating. Even without being a new disorder, the concept of ON makes me argue that when eating becomes a source of suffering, obsession and guilt, we as nutrition and ED experts should look at the issue, with special attention.

# 10 Potential Social Risk Factor for Orthorexia Nervosa: Social Media Use

Pathogenesis of orthorexia nervosa is hitherto an under-researched field; thus, it urgently needs exploration. Unfortunately, no research indicates which factors cause orthorexia nervosa. Therefore, the identification of potential risk factors of orthorexia seems to be warranted (Bundros et al., 2016). The socio-cultural context related to social media's influence on orthorexia nervosa has been explored for several years, mainly using qualitative research methods (e.g. Fixsen, Cheshire & Berry, 2020; Scheiber, Diehl & Karmasin, 2023; Santarossa et al., 2019; Turner & Lefevre, 2017; Valente et al., 2022a, 2022b; White et al., 2021). The popularity of orthorexia nervosa on social media platforms, such as Instagram and Twitter, is perceptible (Valente et al., 2022b). To date, there are over 194,000 posts with the hashtag (#) orthorexia on Instagram (as of 6 December 2023).

Recent evidence has suggested that starting from the second quarter of 2023, internet users spent 6 hours and 41 minutes online daily (this is an increase of 0.15% compared to the preceding quarter) (Statista, 2023). Daily time spent on social media was found to be positively related to orthorexia nervosa. The prevalence of orthorexia nervosa was significantly higher in individuals spending over 60 minutes on social media platforms every day (31%) than in those spending less than 15 minutes a day online (21.8%) (Tarsitano et al., 2022). Although there is some evidence that social media platforms like Instagram and others are linked to mental health problems (e.g. higher levels of depression, eating disorders and related behaviours; Turner & Levefre, 2017), the findings on its relationship with orthorexia nervosa are contradictory. A previous study has suggested that women following accounts focused on a healthy diet on Instagram have a high prevalence of orthorexia nervosa symptoms (measured by the ORTO-15), with higher Instagram use being associated with a greater tendency towards orthorexia nervosa, thus being considered a risk factor for the development of orthorexia nervosa (Turner & Levefre, 2017). Research concerning the social media-based socio-cultural model for orthorexia nervosa (Scheiber, Diehl & Karmasin, 2023) has identified that social media, especially involvement with health and fitness accounts, may be considered a risk factor for orthorexia nervosa. Individuals with higher involvement in health and fitness accounts on social media demonstrated increased symptoms of orthorexia nervosa than those who showed less interest in such content. In addition, they were found to have higher levels of thin-ideal and muscular internalisations, which further contributed to higher levels of orthorexia nervosa symptoms. By contrast, in another study, the use of Instagram was found to be not associated with self-identification of having orthorexia nervosa (Zemlyanskaya, Valente & Syurina, 2022). There are also findings (Santarossa et al., 2019; Valente et al., 2022a) that do not support the notion that Instagram is encouraging orthorexia nervosa. They propose Instagram may be used as a supportive online social network that concentrates on recovery and adopting healthy eating behaviours. Thus, it could be concluded that Instagram and other social media platforms (e.g. Twitter) can be both 'vectors of transmission and recovery' of orthorexia nervosa (Hanganu-Bresch, 2020, p. 316).

# Highlights

- Even though maladaptive preoccupation with healthy eating through strict dietary rules negatively affects mental health, the evidence presented in this chapter suggests that the relationships between orthorexia nervosa and self-esteem, disordered eating and body image are inconclusive. In individuals with orthorexia nervosa, positive self-esteem appears to be due to maintaining a healthy diet and having control over their desires (e.g. Bratman & Knight, 2000; Kinzl et al., 2006), whereas some evidence has suggested lower levels of self-esteem (e.g. Sfeir et al., 2022). Although Bratman (1997) suggested that orthorexia nervosa excludes body image components, some findings provide evidence supporting the hypothesis that there is an association between orthorexia and body image concerns. For instance, individuals with orthorexia nervosa had been profiled as having lower levels of positive body image (body appreciation, appreciation and respect for the body and experience of embodiment) (Anastasiades & Argyrides, 2023) or displayed negative body image components (e.g. Messer et al., 2022). Despite the lack of conclusive results, it is essential to emphasise that some psychological features common to anorexia nervosa and/or obsessive-compulsive disorder have also been found in individuals with orthorexia nervosa (Figure 10.1).

- On the psychological level, certain personality traits were found to be linked to orthorexia nervosa, namely self-oriented, others-oriented and socially prescribed perfectionism (Barnes & Caltabiano, 2017). In addition, individuals with orthorexia nervosa were characterised by high levels of anxiety, avoidant attachment styles and a need for control (Barnes & Caltabiano, 2017). Perceived control, perfectionism and a confirmatory cycle of fear and avoidance were found to be possible key factors in the development and maintenance of orthorexia nervosa (Greville-Harris, Smithson & Karl, 2020). According to the transdiagnostic cognitive behavioural theory of eating disorders (Fairburn, Cooper & Shafran, 2003), perfectionism is an antecedent of disordered eating. It develops and maintains a self-concept focused on appearance (overvaluation of body shape/weight), which is the core psychopathology underlying anorexia nervosa and bulimia nervosa. In the context of orthorexia, perfectionism may cultivate a focused self-concept (i.e. placing overriding importance on a single area of life for self-definition and self-worth; Veale, 2002) on health, which is the core underlying orthorexia nervosa. Moreover, some evidence suggests that

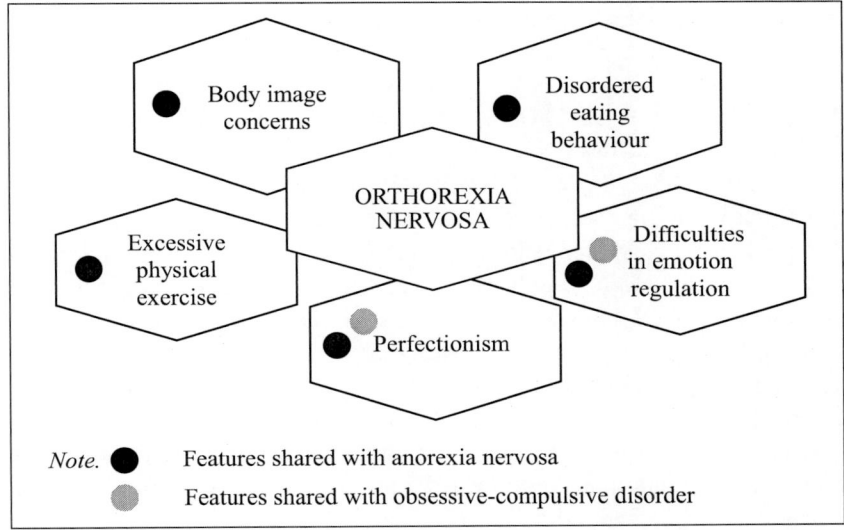

**Figure 10.1** Psychological characteristics of orthorexia nervosa: features shared with anorexia nervosa and obsessive-compulsive disorder based on existing evidence.

orthorexia nervosa symptoms may stem, in part, from having a health-focused self-concept, that is, overvaluing the importance of health for self-definition and self-worth (Tabri, Yung & Elliott, 2022).

• The studies presented thus far provide evidence that individuals with orthorexia nervosa consumed mainly healthy food, followed a strict eating schedule, avoided foods with specific colours, and had a higher tendency to eat the same food every day and to spend a considerable amount of time on the preparation of meals. They considered being overweight more often as a sign of weakness, blamed people for their diseases, and judged people negatively who could not overcome their desires and who did not follow the rules of healthy nutrition (Varga et al., 2014). Orthorexia nervosa is associated with the choice of healthy food (consuming more vegetables, fruits and full grains, whole wheat cereals) as well as with healthy lifestyle characteristics, such as regular sports activity, being on special diets, inclination to persuade others about the importance of a healthy diet, and limited alcohol intake (Varga et al., 2014). As suggested in the previous study (Almeida, Vieira Borba & Santos, 2018), individuals with orthorexia nervosa, apart from preoccupation with restrictions on a healthy diet, may experience physical appearance and exercising issues (e.g. feeling guilty when not doing as much exercise as desired, and missing out on other activities to follow physical training or strict meal schedules).

Diverse motives for excessive physical activity in individuals with orthorexia nervosa have been identified so far: enhancing health (Bratman, 1997; Dunn & Bratman, 2016), subduing a chronic disease (Bratman, 1997), improving both psychological and physical health and social relationships (Oberle, Watkins & Burkot, 2018) as well as enhancing mood, weight control, social desirability and healthy lifestyle (Kiss-Leizer, Tóth-Király & Rigó, 2019).

• Conceivably, in individuals with orthorexia nervosa, healthy nutrition and physical activity may reflect the motivation to reach a healthy lifestyle and to maintain optimal health (Kiss-Leizer, Tóth-Király & Rigó, 2019). It can be assumed that in individuals with orthorexia nervosa, health concern (i.e. achieving optimal health) drives physical exercise (contrary to individuals with anorexia nervosa, in whom weight loss or prevention of weight gain guides excessive exercise) (Oberle, Watkins & Burkot, 2018). It is worth taking into account that in the case of recovery from orthorexia nervosa, excessive exercise activity compensation might occur with increased feelings of losing control of individuals' eating behaviours during treatment (Oberle, Watkins & Burkot, 2018). Because of the relationship of orthorexia nervosa with excessive physical activity, supervised exercise training in patients with orthorexia nervosa could be taken into consideration. A meta-analysis on the effects of supervised exercise training in patients with anorexia nervosa (Ng, Ng & Wong, 2013) demonstrated that two single-group studies demonstrated significant before and after improvement in weight and body fat after supervised exercise training, while pooled randomised controlled trials and quasi-randomised studies showed no significant effect of supervised exercise training on anthropometry. Furthermore, supervised exercise training influenced a decrease in concerns about body weight, shape and depression as well as perception of exercise in patients with anorexia nervosa. This suggests that incorporating a supervised exercise programme into the management of anorexia nervosa may have psychological and physiological benefits (Ng, Ng & Wong, 2013). It would be notable for individuals with orthorexia nervosa to become aware of their non-exercise physical activity (i.e. daily activities that require movement of the human body without planning or strict control of the physical effort made; Bonilla et al., 2023), such as walking, dancing, gardening among many other activities. Perhaps it could help them diminish engagement in purposeful physical activity.

• It has been postulated that exercise addiction should be comprehended as a risk factor for orthorexia nervosa (Strahler, Wachten & Mueller-Alcazar, 2021), while weight manipulation may be a component of orthorexia nervosa, as weight is commonly used as a proxy marker for health in an orthorexic society (Foyster et al., 2023).

• A psychosocial model of orthorexia nervosa (based on a review of risk factors related to orthorexia nervosa) has been previously proposed (McComb & Mills, 2019). The authors hypothesised that the combination of psychological (namely, perfectionism, dieting/restrictive eating, drive for thinness/thin-ideal internalisation, neuroticism, obsessive-compulsive tendencies, current or past eating disorder, fear of losing control, perceived vulnerability) and social factors (namely, living in a culture that stigmatises obesity, having access to organic/clean foods, having higher income, having access to food research/knowledge, having positive reinforcement from others and time for food planning/preparation) can lead to orthorexia nervosa. Glorifying certain dietary practices in social media can reinforce some individuals' beliefs that only 'pure' and 'healthy' food choices are acceptable (Staudacher & Harer, 2018) and that their food intake makes them superior to others. Previous research has established that some individuals with self-identification of having orthorexia nervosa engage in downward comparisons about health and calorie intake with those perceived by them as having less healthy lifestyles, and that brings a sense of superiority to others (Greville-Harris, Smithson & Karl, 2020).

• Given the dominant socio-cultural belief of healthism (the pursuit of health at all costs) and the development of an orthorexic society whereby orthorexic behaviours are normalised and accepted, orthorexia nervosa may be more prevalent in society than previously expected (Foyster et al., 2023). Thus, clinicians should be aware of orthorexic behaviours and consider screening for orthorexia nervosa (Foyster et al., 2023) in individuals with a history of an eating disorder, endurance athletes and/or active individuals (e.g. fitness participants, gym attendees, exercise students), and those who have weight control as well as those with negative body image.

# Part V

# Two Decades of Research on Orthorexia Nervosa

# 11 Orthorexia Nervosa Research in Western Societies

## 11.1 Orthorexia Nervosa in the Non-clinical Samples

### 11.1.1 College and University Students

Orthorexia nervosa is an area of increasing interest in both research and clinical settings. Most of the knowledge about orthorexia nervosa has emerged from studies of non-clinical and at-risk populations and has focused on differential diagnosis. Internationally, most research on orthorexia nervosa has occurred in college and/or university students (e.g. Clifford & Blyth, 2019; Guglielmetti et al., 2022; King & Wengreen, 2023; Rodgers, White & Berry, 2021; Weinstock & Mazzeo, 2022). The research on orthorexia nervosa among students is diverse in terms of the field of study (e.g. dietetics, nutrition, medicine, health science, exercise science), sex and nationality.

**Orthorexia Nervosa Measured by the ORTO-15**

A large number of studies on orthorexia nervosa based on the ORTO-15 and its modification have been conducted among student samples. For instance, a previous study revealed that orthorexia nervosa, in combination with a high level of physical activity, was higher in Swedish male exercise science students than female business students (Malmborg et al., 2017). Contrary, no significant sex differences in the symptomatology of orthorexia nervosa were found in students from the United Kingdom (Clifford & Blyth, 2019) and Poland (Brytek-Matera et al., 2015a), while in Italy (Dell'Osso et al., 2016) and Brazil (Elias, Gomes & Paracampo, 2022), female students were more likely to have orthorexia nervosa in comparison to male students. Turkish students with orthorexia nervosa had a higher habit of reading food labels, including nutrients (e.g. energy, protein, carbohydrate, saturated fat, cholesterol, total fat, fibre and sugar content), nutritional content information, amount of health claim, usage pattern, food additives, nutritional values and brand information compared to students with normal eating behaviour. Additionally, they were more likely to agree with the idea that reading food labels is important for healthy food selection (Yardımcı & Demirer, 2022). So far, one experimental study has been conducted in the field of orthorexia nervosa among university students (Lakritz et al., 2022). This study assessed the association between food and moral attributes by manipulating the food's objective calorie content (kcal/100 g). High-calorie foods were found to be implicitly related to moral impurity. In contrast, low-calorie foods were found to be implicitly linked to moral purity in French students with orthorexia nervosa. The hypothesis that individuals with orthorexia nervosa associate moral attributes with food more strongly than healthy eating groups has not been confirmed in this study (Lakritz et al., 2022).

## Orthorexia Nervosa Measured by the Eating Habits Questionnaire

No significant sex differences in the symptomatology of orthorexia nervosa were found in students in the United States (Oberle, Watkins & Burkot, 2018). Major symptomatology of orthorexia nervosa was found in Lebanese students compared with the Polish and Italian ones (Mahfoud et al., 2023) and in Polish students compared to Italian ones (Brytek-Matera et al., 2022). The previous study (Weinstock & Mazzeo, 2022) revealed that the diet individuals follow does impact how others view them. US college students ascribed the most negative attributes to individuals with orthorexia nervosa and an intermittent fasting diet as well. In comparison, those adhering to a clean eating diet were viewed most favourably. The type of diet, namely vegetarian or vegan diet, and the frequency of diet, namely having followed one diet in one's lifetime, was related to orthorexia nervosa in Italian students (Novara et al., 2022b).

## Orthorexia Nervosa Measured by the Düsseldorf Orthorexia Scale

A recent study revealed that orthorexia nervosa was positively associated with disordered eating symptoms (e.g. restrictive eating, binge eating and purging behaviours, willingness to lose weight, ruminating, worrying about weight and body shape, engaging in intense physical exercise to lose weight), obsessive-compulsive symptoms and depressive symptoms in Italian students (Cerolini et al., 2022). In Brazilian undergraduate and graduate college students, orthorexia nervosa was linked to attitudes, feelings and behaviours related to eating pathology (especially dieting, bulimia and food preoccupation) and obsessive-compulsive symptoms as well (Souza et al., 2021). In Spanish students, orthorexia nervosa was also positively related to eating disorder symptoms (drive for thinness, body dissatisfaction, bulimia, effectiveness, perfectionism, interoceptive awareness, asceticism, impulse regulation and social insecurity) (Parra-Fernández et al., 2019).

## Orthorexia Nervosa Measured by the Teruel Orthorexia Scale

Previous evidence has suggested that women are more likely to have orthorexia nervosa than men. In contrast, no significant sex differences in terms of healthy orthorexia were observed in the general population in Brazil (Roberto da Silva et al., 2021). Healthy orthorexia and orthorexia nervosa revealed opposite patterns of correlations with disordered eating behaviours and obsessive-compulsive symptoms in the general population in France (Lasson et al., 2023) and in the United States (Zickgraf & Barrada, 2022). The positive association of orthorexia nervosa with social appearance anxiety was found in the general population in Brazil (Roberto da Silva et al., 2021).

The psychological research's over-reliance on convenience samples of undergraduate students has been a topic of concern and discussion over the past two decades (Wild, Kyröläinen & Kuperman, 2022). Student samples (college and/or university students) predominate in psychological and cross-cultural studies with adults (Foot & Sanford, 2004; Hanel & Vione, 2016). A previous meta-analysis of scientific data (Arnett, 2008) revealed that in 67% of American studies published in *The Journal of Personality and Social Psychology* in 2007, the samples comprised undergraduate psychology students. The percentage of psychology student samples in non-American studies was 80%. Using student samples in psychological research concerns issues related to representativeness, generalisability, and comparability of results (Hanel & Vione, 2016). Recent evidence has demonstrated that the undergraduate student population is unrepresentative of the general population (Wild, Kyröläinen & Kuperman, 2022). Although collecting normative population-wide data is an expensive and time-consuming process (Wild, Kyröläinen & Kuperman, 2022), we cannot have a tendency to make conclusions about human nature based on samples taken solely from undergraduate students. Therefore, we need research across diverse populations to address explicitly the question of the representativeness of samples and generalisability in study samples.

## 11.1.2 General Population

Many studies have been conducted on specific groups of subjects selected from the general population (with a predominance of the ORTO-15 use):

- adolescents (Azzi et al., 2023; D'Urso et al., 2023; Mhanna et al., 2022; Rogoza et al., 2021; Samaha et al., 2022; Yakın et al., 2022; Yurtdaş-Depboylu, Kaner & Özçakal, 2022),
- athletes (Bert et al., 2019; D'Urso et al., 2023; Foyster et al., 2023; Martinovic et al., 2022; Özdengül et al., 2021; Paludo et al., 2022; Segura-Garcia et al., 2012; Surała et al., 2020; Toti et al., 2022; Uriegas et al., 2021),
- dancers (Athanasaki et al., 2023) and/or performance artists (Aksoydan & Camci, 2009),
- dieticians (Alvarenga et al., 2012; Asil & Sürücüoğlu, 2015; Caferoglu & Toklu, 2022; Kinzl et al., 2006; Souza et al., 2021; Tremelling et al., 2017),
- gym members (Almeida et al., 2018; Mavrandrea & Gonidakis, 2022; Rudolph, 2018),

- health professionals (Douma, Valente & Syurina, 2021; Gramaglia et al., 2022; Reynolds & McMahon, 2019; Ryman et al., 2019; Sanzari & Hormes, 2023; Vandereycken, 2011),
- individuals following plant-based diets (Albery et al., 2022; Barthels, Meyer & Pietrowsky, 2018; Brytek-Matera, 2020a, 2020b, 2021b; Brytek-Matera et al., 2019; Çiçekoğlu & Tunçay, 2018; Kalika, Egan & Mantzios, 2022; Parra-Fernández et al., 2020; Reynolds et al., 2023),
- pregnant women (Gerontidis et al., 2022; Taştekin Ouyaba & Çiçekoğlu Öztürk, 2022),
- premenopausal, perimenopausal and postmenopausal women (Khalil et al., 2022; Raynal et al., 2022),
- youth female soccer players (Paludo et al., 2023).

**Orthorexia Nervosa Measured by the Eating Habits Questionnaire**

A recent study (Bali et al., 2023) demonstrated that Greek women and men do not differ in terms of orthorexia nervosa. Orthorexia nervosa was more strongly linked with eating disorder pathology than with obsessive-compulsive and depressive symptomatology and personality traits among the Greek general population (Bali et al., 2023). While, in the general population in the United States, orthorexia nervosa was more strongly associated with severe restricting for thinness and binge/purge symptoms than with avoidant/restrictive food intake disorder symptoms as well as moderately positively associated with fruit/vegetable proportion and moderately negatively associated with discretionary food intake (snack/dessert proportion) (Zickgraf, Ellis & Essayli, 2019). The positive association of orthorexia nervosa with cognitive restraint, uncontrolled eating and emotional eating was observed in the Polish general population (Brytek-Matera, Plasonja & Décamps, 2020), whereas in the Australian general population, orthorexia nervosa symptoms were most strongly associated with eating pathology, as opposed to depression, anxiety and obsessive-compulsive tendencies (Walker-Swanton, Hay & Conti, 2020).

Previous research has established that individuals following a vegetarian diet report more orthorexic behaviour related to knowledge of healthy eating, problems associated with healthy eating and feeling positively about healthy eating than those who follow an omnivorous diet (Brytek-Matera, 2020a, 2020b). Moreover, individuals following a vegan diet were more likely to develop cognitive orthorexic behaviours if they adhered to a meat-free diet for health reasons (Brytek-Matera et al., 2019). Following a plant-based diet could prompt more focus on the quality of food and food consumption, which may indicate that individuals following a vegetarian diet are more likely to display orthorexia nervosa (Brytek-Matera, 2020a, 2020b; Brytek-Matera et al., 2019).

## Orthorexia Nervosa Measured by the Düsseldorf Orthorexia Scale

No significant sex differences in orthorexia nervosa were found in the Italian general population (Aloi et al., 2023). Meanwhile, in the Portuguese general population, women presented significantly higher orthorexic behaviours than men (Ferreira & Coimbra, 2021). Moreover, perimenopausal women and postmenopausal women were more prone to orthorexia nervosa than pre-menopausal women. The prevalence of orthorexia nervosa was 6.4%, 4.6% and 2.7% in perimenopausal, postmenopausal and premenopausal women, respectively (Raynal et al., 2022). It has also been demonstrated that individuals following plant-based diets (vegetarian or vegan diet) displayed higher levels of orthorexic eating behaviour and were at higher risk of developing orthorexia nervosa compared with those who did not follow a particular diet (Barthels, Meyer & Pietrowsky, 2018; Chard et al., 2019; Lasson, Barthels & Raynal, 2021). Additionally, individuals showing restrained eating behaviour mainly for ethical reasons or to lose weight presented more orthorexic eating behaviour than those who did not limit their food intake (Barthels, Meyer & Pietrowsky, 2018).

Thus far, previous studies indicated that orthorexia nervosa is positively associated with psychopathology symptomatology (anxiety, depression and stress) and shame (external and internal) in the Portuguese general population (Ferreira & Coimbra, 2021), disgust sensitivity in the Italian general population (Aloi et al., 2023), depression, stress, somatoform symptoms and eating disorder symptoms in the German general population (Greetfeld et al., 2021) as well as with (rigid, self-critical and narcissistic) perfectionism in the general population in the United Kingdom (Miley et al., 2022). However, only the rigid perfectionism dimension predicted a significant increase in orthorexic eating behaviours in this group. In addition, higher awareness of eating during eating occurrences (a facet of mindful eating) was related to reduced orthorexic eating behaviours (Miley et al., 2022). Orthorexia nervosa was positively related to depression and anxiety symptoms, body image dissatisfaction and age, and negatively to self-esteem and body mass index in women in France aged between 30 and 71 years (Raynal et al., 2022). Orthorexia nervosa was linked to low levels of self-compassion and high levels of restrained eating in individuals following a vegan diet. Furthermore, self-compassion mediated the relationship between restrictive eating and orthorexia nervosa in this group (Kalika, Egan & Mantzios, 2022).

### Orthorexia Nervosa Measured by the Teruel Orthorexia Scale

Healthy orthorexia was found to be negatively and significantly linked to somatisation, depression and anxiety in the general population in Italy (Falgares et al., 2023) and unrelated to both eating disorders and obsessive-compulsive symptoms in the general population in Italy (Falgares et al., 2023), whereas orthorexia nervosa was positively and significantly associated with somatisation, depression and anxiety (Falgares et al., 2023; Sezer Katar, Şahin & Kurtoğlu, 2023) as well as with obsessive-compulsive symptomatology and eating disorders symptoms in the general population in Italy (Falgares et al., 2023) and in the United States (Chace & Kluck, 2022). A positive association was also found between orthorexia nervosa and health anxiety, concern over mistakes (the experience of negative emotions as a result of mistakes, equating mistakes to failure, and belief that mistakes cause a loss of respect), negative affect and dysphoric body image emotions in a US sample (Chace & Kluck, 2022). Orthorexia nervosa was also related to increased obsessive-compulsive symptoms, perfectionism and cognitive biases (i.e. slowed disengagement) in individuals adhering to a vegetarian or vegan diet in the United Kingdom (Albery et al., 2022).

### Orthorexia Nervosa Measured by the Orthorexia Nervosa Inventory

Recent evidence suggests that orthorexia nervosa is associated with psychosocial impairment due to eating disorders features, the core features of anorexia nervosa and bulimia nervosa and obsessive-compulsive symptoms in the general Italian population (Zagaria et al., 2023).

It has resulted from a variety of studies that the at-risk population for orthorexia nervosa include college and university students, especially in dietetics and nutrition, individuals following a plant-based diet and athletes. In some studies, gym members, (peri- and post-) menopausal women and adolescents were also considered to be at risk for developing the condition. In the majority of cross-sectional studies, the occurrence of eating disorder symptoms or a previous eating disorder history, obsessive-compulsive symptoms and/or depression has consistently been demonstrated as conditions increasing the risk of developing orthorexia nervosa (McComb & Mills, 2019). However, considering the disadvantages of cross-sectional studies (e.g. the lack of the dimension of time and causal relationships and the exhibition of recall bias), these findings must be interpreted carefully.

## 11.1.3 Health Professionals' Perspectives on Orthorexia Nervosa

Having expertise in orthorexia nervosa is vital to providing professional help to individuals with this condition; by contrast, its lack could inhibit greater involvement in care and treatment (Lester, Tritter & Sorohan, 2005). The lack of knowledge about orthorexia nervosa was emphasised by almost 10% of professionals in the field of eating disorders in Belgium more than 10 years ago (Vandereycken, 2011). Since then, relatively little research has sought health professionals' opinions on orthorexia nervosa. There has been research conducted in Australia and New Zealand (Reynolds & McMahon, 2019), the Netherlands (Ryman et al., 2019), Italy (Gramaglia et al., 2022) and the United States (Sanzari & Hormes, 2023) (Table 11.1). Many medical, psychological and nutritional specialists stated that their knowledge regarding orthorexia nervosa is sufficient (Barthels et al., 2019). The existing findings indicated that the overwhelming majority of health professionals with experience working clinically with eating disorders indicated that orthorexia nervosa should be included as a diagnosis in the upcoming version(s) of the DSM as a distinct, clinically recognised disorder. Health professionals who spend more time conducting clinical work were more likely to endorse orthorexia nervosa as a discrete diagnosis compared to those who reported spending more time on research (Sanzari & Hormes, 2023). According to the vast majority of health professionals, orthorexia nervosa fits within the DSM category of 'Eating and Feeding Disorders'. Their opinion was based on their clinical experience with individuals suffering from orthorexia nervosa-like symptoms (Sanzari & Hormes, 2023).

Table 11.1 Health professionals' opinions on orthorexia nervosa as a disordered eating pattern: the percentage of the affirmative answers

| Opinion | Netherlands (N = 160) | Italy (N = 343) | United States (N = 100) |
|---|---|---|---|
| Regarding orthorexia nervosa as a distinct clinical diagnosis | 77.5% | Not applicable | 71.9% |
| Including orthorexia nervosa in a future version(s) of the DSM | Not applicable | 68.5% | 71.9% |
| Having experience of working with individuals who fulfilled the diagnostic criteria for orthorexia nervosa | 63.1% | 58.9% | 78.1%* |
| Fitting orthorexia nervosa within the DSM category of 'Eating and Feeding Disorders' | 74.2% | 82.1% | 94.8% |

Table 11.1 (cont.)

| Opinion | Netherlands (N = 160) | Italy (N = 343) | United States (N = 100) |
|---|---|---|---|
| Including exercise-related symptoms in diagnostic criteria of orthorexia nervosa | 68.8% | 56.8% | 62.1% |
| Similarity of treatment of orthorexia nervosa to the treatment of eating disorders | Not applicable | 60.9% | Not applicable |

Note: * Criteria proposed by Dunn and Bratman (2016).

Health professionals reported that socio-cultural factors have considerable influence on the development of ON, namely the diet and weight loss industry and the perceptions that biological/organic/vegan and low fat/low carb/gluten-free food are the healthiest (Gramaglia et al., 2022; Sanzari & Hormes, 2023). Other possible contributing factors, such as dietary trends, health misinformation, 'fitspiration', social media, thin ideals, social pressures, and lack of control in other aspects of life, were also suggested (Reynolds & McMahon, 2019).

Individuals with orthorexia nervosa search for professional help and information on ways to change their maladaptive eating behaviour. Over a decade ago, almost 67% of professionals in the field of eating disorders had experience consulting patients with orthorexia nervosa (Vandereycken, 2011). Nowadays, over two-thirds of German nutritionists declare that they have been consulted by at least one individual with symptoms resembling orthorexic eating behaviour during the last 12 months (Barthels et al., 2019) and over three-quarters of health specialists in the United States (Sanzari & Hormes, 2023) and 85% in Australia and New Zealand (Reynolds & McMahon, 2019) have experience in the everyday professional routine of specialists with working with individuals with orthorexia nervosa. Until now, no research has encompassed the dual perspectives of health professionals and patients with orthorexia nervosa. Thus, combined focus groups (health professionals and patients) helped highlight their needs and expectations.

## 11.2 Orthorexia Nervosa in the Clinical Samples

A large and growing body of literature has been published on orthorexia nervosa among the general population. In contrast, an inconsiderable amount of research has been conducted among patients with different mental disorders and conditions. PubMed® database was used in a literature search, resulting in six empirical research studies on orthorexia nervosa in patients with eating disorders, four empirical research studies on orthorexia nervosa in patients with obsessive-compulsive disorder, one empirical research on orthorexia nervosa in patients with somatic symptom disorder and one case report of orthorexia nervosa in a patient with depression.

## 11.2.1 Patients with Eating Disorders

The findings of the first paper in this research field (Segura-Garcia et al., 2015; see Table 11.2) revealed that patients with a diagnosis of anorexia nervosa or bulimia nervosa presented higher levels of orthorexia nervosa than the healthy control group (high school and college students). The levels of orthorexia nervosa were lower in patients with eating disorders at the time of the first visit to the outpatient clinic than after a minimum of three years from the end of treatment. The findings also indicated that the frequency of orthorexia nervosa increases over time among patients with eating disorders (28% at first visit versus 53% after treatment). Based on a transdiagnostic approach, the authors

Table 11.2 The summary of existing studies on orthorexia nervosa in patients with eating disorders*

| Authors (years) | Sample | Orthorexia nervosa: method mean ± standard deviation | Differences between samples in terms of orthorexia nervosa |
|---|---|---|---|
| Barthels et al., 2017 | 29 female inpatients with anorexia nervosa with pronounced orthorexic eating behaviour (ANO+): $M_{age} = 19.97 \pm 4.52$ 13 female inpatients with anorexia nervosa with low orthorexic eating behaviour (ANO-): $M_{age} = 23.85 \pm 10.13$ 30 female healthy individuals (HI): $M_{age} = 22.10 \pm 7.43$ | Düsseldorf Orthorexia Scale $M_{ANO+} = 32.83 \pm 4.41$ $M_{ANO-} = 32.08 \pm 5.45$ $M_{HI} = 19.03 \pm 4.53$ | ANO+ > HI $(p < 0.001)$ ANO- > HI $(p < 0.044)$ |

Table 11.2 (cont.)

| Authors (years) | Sample | Orthorexia nervosa: method mean ± standard deviation | Differences between samples in terms of orthorexia nervosa |
|---|---|---|---|
| Busatta et al., 2022 | 30 female patients with eating disorders (EDs) 30 female student dietitians 30 female healthy individuals | ORTO-15 $M_{EDs} = 33.23 \pm 5.58$ $M_{SD} = 38.23 \pm 3.28$ $M_{HI} = 38.47 \pm 3.64$ | EDs > SD $(p < 0.001)$ EDs > HI $(p < 0.001)$ |
| Gramaglia et al., 2017 | 23 female patients with anorexia nervosa (AN) from Italy: $M_{age} = 30.39$ 35 female patients with anorexia nervosa from Poland: 83.3% women: $M_{age} = 22.97$ 39 female healthy individuals (HI) from Italy: $M_{age} = 34.41$ 39 female healthy individuals from Poland: $M_{age} = 23.00$ | ORTO-15 $M_{AN\_Italy} = 37.21 \pm 1.15$ $M_{AN\_Poland} = 34.37 \pm 0.83$ $M_{HI\_Italy} = 39.41 \pm 0.50$ $M_{HI\_Poland} = 35.36 \pm 0.58$ | $AN_{Italy} > HI_{Italy}$ $(p = 0.049)$ $AN_{Italy} < AN_{Poland}$ $(p = 0.044)$ $HI_{Italy} < HI_{Poland}$ $(p = 0.001)$ |
| Hessler-Kaufmann et al. 2021 | 218 inpatients with anorexia nervosa (AN): $M_{age} = 22.7 \pm 8.75$ 63 inpatients with bulimia nervosa (BN) $M_{age} = 24.2 \pm 9.89$ 315 inpatients with recurrent depressive disorder (DD): $M_{age} = 45.3 \pm 15.3$ 228 inpatients with depressive episode (DE) | Düsseldorf Orthorexia Scale AN $M_{Admission} = 27.9 \pm 7.97$ $M_{Discharge} = 20.7 \pm 7.20$ BN $M_{Admission} = 25.3 \pm 7.30$ $M_{Discharge} = 17.7 \pm 6.37$ DD $M_{Admission} = 16.1 \pm 5.17$ $M_{Discharge} = 15.8 \pm 4.97$ | $AN_{Admission} > AN_{Discharge}$ $(p < 0.001)$ $BN_{Admission} > BN_{Discharge}$ $(p < 0.001)$ Orthorexia nervosa Remained unchanged from admission to discharge in the other diagnostic groups $(ps > 0.28)$ |

Table 11.2 (cont.)

| Authors (years) | Sample | Orthorexia nervosa: method mean ± standard deviation | Differences between samples in terms of orthorexia nervosa |
|---|---|---|---|
| | $M_{age} = 39.6 \pm 16.2$ 152 inpatients with obsessive-compulsive disorder (OCD): $M_{age} = 33.1 \pm 14.9$ 78 inpatients with trauma-related disorders (TD): $M_{age} = 39.0 \pm 14.0$ 60 inpatients with phobic disorders (PD): $M_{age} = 26.9 \pm 13.1$ 53 inpatients with somatoform disorders (SD): $M_{age} = 45.9 \pm 16.2$ | DE $M_{Admission} = 15.3 \pm 5.07$ $M_{Discharge} = 14.7 \pm 5.15$ OCD $M_{Admission} = 15.2 \pm 5.49$ $M_{Discharge} = 14.8 \pm 5.54$ TD $M_{Admission} = 16.6 \pm 5.52$ $M_{Discharge} = 16.6 \pm 5.02$ PD $M_{Admission} = 14.4 \pm 5.20$ $M_{Discharge} = 14.2 \pm 6.06$ SD $M_{Admission} = 15.0 \pm 3.93$ $M_{Discharge} = 14.2 \pm 3.66$ | |
| Segura-Garcia et al., 2015 | 32 female patients with eating disorders (EDs) Admission (A): $M_{age} = 17.7 \pm 3.5$ After treatment (AT): $M_{age} = 22.2 \pm 3.4$ 32 female healthy individuals: (HI): $M_{age} = 21.9 \pm 3.4$ | ORTO-15 $M_{EDsA} = 37.4 \pm 3.7$ $M_{EDsAT} = 35.2 \pm 4.7$ $M_{HI} = 41.8 \pm 3.3$ | $EDs_A < EDs_{AT}$ $(p = 0.05)$ $EDs_{AT} > CG$ $(p < 0.001)$ |

* Note. One existing study (Brytek-Matera et al., 2015b) was not included in Table 11.2 because in this study sample was only composed of patients with eating disorders. The comparison between samples (presented in Table 11.2) was therefore impossible.

(Segura-Garcia et al., 2015) have proposed that if orthorexia nervosa could be considered as an altered behaviour within the spectrum of eating disorders, its changes over time could be interpreted as an evolution of the illness, that is, the migration towards less severe forms of eating pathology: from eating disorders (preoccupation with food quantity) to orthorexia nervosa (preoccupation with food quality). Other results (Brytek-Matera et al., 2015b) demonstrated that higher levels of eating disorder pathology, weight concern, appearance orientation (i.e. the extent of investment in own appearance) and health orientation (i.e. the extent of investment in a healthy lifestyle) predicted orthorexia nervosa (assessed by the ORTO-15) among patients with eating disorders ($N$ = 52). The findings of a previous cross-cultural study (Gramaglia et al., 2017) demonstrated that patients with anorexia nervosa from Italy had higher levels of orthorexia nervosa than their compatriots from the healthy group but lower levels of orthorexia nervosa in comparison with patients with anorexia nervosa from Poland. The authors (Gramaglia et al., 2017) have drawn attention to the fact that these differences are likely due to culture-related discrepancies in the approach to food and health concepts. The Italian culture has a vibrant tradition in nutrition, and the Mediterranean diet has been acknowledged as an intangible cultural heritage by UNESCO since 2010 (Colao et al., 2022). It is characterised by a healthy nutritional model and has long been recognised for its benefits for overall health, whereas in Poland, in the recent decade, good consumer eating behaviours and habits have gained greater popularity (e.g. checking the composition of foodstuffs), and healthy eating has become the most important among various activities to improve one's health. This may explain the high levels of orthorexia nervosa in the Polish sample. In another study (Barthels et al., 2017), patients with anorexia nervosa with pronounced orthorexic eating behaviour have higher levels of basic psychological needs in the context of eating and dieting concerning autonomy and competence, as well as the dimension of the body image related to self-aggrandisement than patients with anorexia nervosa with low orthorexic eating behaviour. In addition, patients with anorexia nervosa with pronounced orthorexic eating behaviour report eating healthy food regardless of calorie content (low-calorie content and high-calorie content) more frequently than the second clinical sample. Both groups of patients with anorexia nervosa report a higher drive for thinness compared to women with normal eating behaviour. In addition, patients with anorexia nervosa with pronounced orthorexic eating behaviour displayed lower levels of vitality, self-acceptance, sexual satisfaction (three dimensions of body image) and relatedness (one of the basic psychological needs in the context of eating and dieting), and higher levels of competence than the control group. The authors (Barthels et al., 2017) assume that orthorexic eating behaviour might serve as a coping strategy for patients with anorexia nervosa and might help them to recover from their eating disorder. In other words, orthorexia nervosa appears to be a strategy for compensating food restriction in anorexia nervosa, allowing patients to eat more while still being highly selective with their choices as well as maintaining control over their eating behaviour (Barthels et al., 2017). The prevalence of and changes of orthorexia nervosa (assessed by the Düsseldorf Orthorexia Scale) during disorder-specific treatment in a large sample of inpatients with mental disorders, including eating disorders, depressive disorders, obsessive-compulsive disorder, somatoform, and anxiety disorders, were investigated (Hessler-Kaufmann et al., 2021). The prevalence of orthorexia nervosa was higher in patients with eating disorders than in all other groups and ranged between 7.7% (patients with bulimia nervosa at discharge) and 48% (patients with anorexia nervosa at admission) at both admission and discharge, whereas in all other groups, its prevalence ranged between 0% (patients with somatoform disorders at admission and discharge) and 3.7% (patients with obsessive-compulsive disorder at discharge) at both admission and discharge. In addition, in patients with eating disorders, orthorexia nervosa decreased during eating disorder-specific treatment (while there was no change in the other patient groups). The authors (Hessler-Kaufmann et al., 2021) suggest that orthorexia nervosa may represent a phenomenological subtype of a restrictive eating disorder (i.e. part of the eating disorder spectrum) and no distinct clinical entity. Orthorexic tendencies, however, might still precede an eating disorder and later be reflected in its symptoms. Recently, a cross-sectional study (Busatta et al., 2022) found that patients with eating disorders demonstrated higher levels of orthorexia nervosa than both student dietitians and healthy control groups. Moreover, in patients with eating disorders, orthorexia nervosa was moderately associated with more severe eating disorder psychopathology, indicating that orthorexia nervosa is already present in the acute phase of eating disorders (Busatta et al., 2022).

## 11.2.2 Patients with Obsessive-Compulsive Disorder

The first research demonstrated no evidence of a difference between patients with a diagnosis of obsessive-compulsive disorder and those with a diagnosis of generalised anxiety disorder and panic disorder concerning orthorexia nervosa, suggesting that orthorexia nervosa is not specifically associated with any of these disorders (Poyraz et al., 2015; see Table 11.3). Recent findings revealed that outpatients with obsessive-compulsive disorder have lower levels of orthorexia nervosa than healthy individuals who exercise regularly. No evidence of a difference between outpatients with obsessive-compulsive disorder and healthy individuals who did not exercise concerning orthorexia nervosa was found (Yılmaz et al., 2020). In outpatients with obsessive-compulsive disorder, orthorexia nervosa was solely weakly associated with higher levels of disordered eating behaviours. This assumes that orthorexia nervosa is more related to eating disorders than to obsessive-compulsive disorder (Yılmaz et al., 2020). In the other study (Vaccari et al., 2021), no evidence of the differences between patients diagnosed with obsessive-compulsive disorder and patients with a

Table 11.3 The summary of existing studies on orthorexia nervosa in patients with obsessive-compulsive disorder*

| Authors (years) | Sample | Orthorexia nervosa: method mean ± standard deviation | Differences in terms of orthorexia nervosa |
|---|---|---|---|
| Poyraz et al., 2015 | 49 patients with obsessive-compulsive disorder (OCD): 73.46% women $M_{age} = 31.37 \pm 10.97$ 44 patients with panic disorder (PD): 68.18% women $M_{age} = 35.03 \pm 9.58$ 37 patients with generalised anxiety disorder (GAD): 83.78% women $M_{age} = 33.43 \pm 9.96$ | ORTO-11 $M_{OCD} = 28.4 \pm 5.76$ $M_{PD} = 28.4 \pm 5.69$ $M_{GAD} = 28.0 \pm 7.30$ | There is no evidence of a difference between the three groups of patients ($p = 0.948$) |
| Vaccari et al., 2021 | 50 patients diagnosed with obsessive-compulsive disorder (OCD), 32 % of women $M_{age} = 38.3 \pm 12.7$ 42 patients with a diagnosis of anxiety-depressive spectrum disorder (A-DSD): 83.3% of women $M_{age} = 46.2 \pm 13.7$ 236 individuals with no psychiatric morbidity (NPM): 57.2% of women $M_{age} = 34.5 \pm 13.5$ | ORTO-15 $M_{OCD} = 36.8 \pm 5.5$ $M_{A-DSD} = 38.1 \pm 5.1$ $M_{NPM} = 38.1 \pm 3.7$ | There is no evidence of a difference between the three groups (n.s.) |

**Table 11.3 (cont.)**

| Authors (years) | Sample | Orthorexia nervosa: method mean ± standard deviation | Differences in terms of orthorexia nervosa |
|---|---|---|---|
| Yılmaz et al., 2020 | 63 outpatients with obsessive-compulsive disorder (OCD): 63.5% women $M_{age} = 34.69 \pm 10.49$ 63 healthy individuals who exercised regularly (HE+): 55.6% of women $M_{age} = 29.00 \pm 7.84$ 63 healthy individuals who did not exercise (HE-): 55.6% women $M_{age} = 32.74 \pm 12.58$ | ORTO-11 $M_{OCD} = 28.51 \pm 5.61$ $M_{HE+} = 25.70 \pm 4.45$ $M_{HE-} = 29.59 \pm 3.45$ | HE+ > OCD HE+ > HE- $(p < 0.001)$ |

* Note. One existing study (Hessler-Kaufmann et al., 2021) was not included in Table 11.3 because in this study the differences between different diagnostic groups (including patients with obsessive-compulsive disorder) in the prevalence of orthorexic tendencies at admission and their change during disorder-specific treatment was assessed (please see Table 7.1). The comparison between samples (presented in Table 11.3) was therefore impossible.

diagnosis of other psychiatric conditions (anxiety or depressive disorders) and individuals with no psychiatric morbidity concerning orthorexia nervosa was found. In addition, individuals with or without orthorexia nervosa did not differ in terms of symptoms of obsessive-compulsive disorder. Recently, orthorexic tendencies have been found to remain unchanged from admission to discharge in patients with obsessive-compulsive disorder (Hessler-Kaufmann et al., 2021).

### 11.2.3 Patients with Mental Disorders: Somatic Symptom Disorder and Depression

Some researchers have investigated the possible link between orthorexia nervosa and other mental disorders. The recent findings (Barthels et al., 2021) have suggested that patients with somatoform disorders ($N = 31$) report significantly slightly higher levels of orthorexia nervosa than healthy adults, which, however, remain markedly lower than in patients with eating disorders. In addition, orthorexia nervosa was moderately associated with healthy habits and somatisation in eating in those patients. Orthorexia nervosa does not seem to be closely related to behavioural, cognitive, perceptual or affective aspects of somatoform disorders, possibly indicating a slight role within this disorder (Barthels et al.,

2021). The only existing case report has described the clinical and follow-up findings of an 18-year-old woman with orthorexia nervosa comorbid with major depressive disorder treated with mirtazapine (Lopes et al., 2020). The patient had a 12-month history of obsessional thoughts and behaviours related to her diet, including spending several hours a day studying food elements, becoming obsessional for selective healthy eating habits, eating 'clean food' and eating only self-made meals. She progressively suppressed all foods with sugar (including sodas and soft drinks) and fried and processed foods (including fried chips, popcorn and 'fast food'). She banned red meat and certain complex carbohydrates from her diet and preferred vegetables, fruits, fish, dry fruits, berries and white meat (only sporadically). She became more socially isolated. The patient lost approximately 15 kilograms in 12 months (body mass index of 16.2 kg/m$^2$). She denied a fear of being fat or a disturbed body image, episodes of compulsive eating, purgative/compensatory behaviours, amenorrhea or irregular menstrual cycles. The patient met the current diagnostic criteria for orthorexia nervosa (Dunn & Bratman, 2016; Moroze et al., 2015). Orthorexia nervosa preceded the onset of depressive symptomatology. Treatment with mirtazapine for 11 months (ranging from 7.5 mg to 30 mg every night at bedtime; being chosen due to its well-established efficacy on depression and anxiety symptoms) resulted in the resolution of the depression symptoms as well as remission of the obsessional thoughts and behaviour related to healthy eating and an improvement and maintenance of weight gain (body mass index of 19.29 kg/m$^2$). This case report highlights the possible usefulness of mirtazapine as a treatment option for patients with orthorexia nervosa (Lopes et al., 2020). However, the effectiveness of this pharmacological intervention should be assessed in randomised controlled trials.

Single clinical cases have also been described in the literature. One case presented a 33-year-old woman with orthorexia nervosa, whose orthorexic eating behaviour represented a prodrome for the development of paranoid schizophrenia (Saddichha et al., 2012). The patient had a 12-month history of paranoid ideation, bizarre delusions and social withdrawal, which had been preceded by seven years of having pursued an exclusive diet of only fresh fruits and vegetables and raw eggs. Another case report (Rania et al., 2021) revealed that patients who were diagnosed with a prior psychiatric disorder, that is, obsessive-compulsive disorder, bulimia nervosa, illness anxiety disorder, paranoid personality trait and a psychotic disorder not otherwise specified, later developed symptoms suggestive of orthorexia nervosa (assessed by the ORTO-15), suggesting the possibility that these disorders may be related to a later onset of orthorexia nervosa (Rania et al., 2021). However, there is no certainty that these cases should be treated as re-exacerbations of the primary disorders with a different pathological content.

# 12 Research on Orthorexia Nervosa in Non-Western Societies Using the Example of East Asian Countries

Orthorexia nervosa has been poorly studied among adults in East Asia, and there is scant information available on the correlates of orthorexia nervosa in non-Western cultures. To the best of the author's knowledge, four studies were carried out in Mainland China (He et al., 2019, 2021; Li et al., 2022; Zhou et al., 2020), and one case report (Park et al., 2011) and one empirical study (Cho & Hyun, 2020) have been conducted in South Korea. So far, no studies have been published in English on orthorexia nervosa among adults living in Hong Kong, Japan, Macau, Mongolia, North Korea and Taiwan. One case report describing a 13-year-old Japanese girl diagnosed with orthorexia nervosa has been recently published (Yoshimura et al., 2023).

## 12.1 Mainland China

The first published study, conducted among 1,075 university students (52.7% women; $M_{age} = 20.11 \pm 1.01$ years) (He et al., 2019), revealed that the prevalence of orthorexia nervosa (assessed by the Düsseldorf Orthorexia Scale) was 7.8%, whereas 18.2% of students were classified as being at risk of orthorexia nervosa. Moreover, men displayed a significantly higher prevalence rate of orthorexia nervosa than women (10.6% versus 5.3%). Orthorexia nervosa has been found to have a strong positive association with inflexible and rigid eating rules, a weak positive association with cognitive restraint and a weak negative association with uncontrolled eating. The relationships between orthorexia nervosa and emotional eating and body mass index were not significant. Other findings conducted among 418 university students (52.39% women; $M_{age} = 20.00 \pm 1.1$ years) (Zhou et al., 2020) revealed that individuals with higher levels of orthorexia nervosa (assessed by the Orthorexia Nervosa Scale) reported significantly higher obsessive-compulsive and anxiety symptoms compared to those without orthorexia nervosa. No evidence of a difference between women and men concerning symptoms of orthorexia nervosa over the past six months was found; however, women had higher levels of severe orthorexia nervosa symptoms over the past week than men. The severity of orthorexia nervosa symptoms was positively associated with obsessive-compulsive disorder symptoms and anxiety symptoms (moderate correlations), as well as being positively associated with depressive symptoms and fear of negative evaluation (weak correlations). Symptoms of orthorexia nervosa were related to all variables except depressive symptoms. One study on orthorexia nervosa (He et al., 2021) was conducted among the elderly in China ($N$ = 313; $M$ = 67.90 ± 7.94 years; 51.8% women). These findings revealed that 19.5% were identified as having orthorexia nervosa (assessed by the Düsseldorf Orthorexia Scale). Older women and men with orthorexia nervosa had significantly higher levels of physical activity, life satisfaction, consumption of fruit and vegetables, body appreciation and functionality appreciation than those without orthorexia nervosa. Moreover, there was a weak positive association between orthorexia nervosa and physical activity, fruit and vegetable consumption, body appreciation, functionality appreciation and life satisfaction, providing initial support for a positive psychology perspective of orthorexia nervosa in this group. Thus, according to the authors (He et al., 2021), orthorexia nervosa in the elderly in China might not be viewed as a form of disordered eating but can be protective and beneficial. A negative association was found between orthorexia nervosa and body dissatisfaction, suggesting a protective role of orthorexia nervosa in negative body image in the elderly. Similarly, orthorexia nervosa was not correlated with traditional disordered eating symptomology, suggesting a dissociation with other disordered eating (He et al., 2021). The associations of orthorexia nervosa with positive body image and life satisfaction (He et al., 2021) could suggest orthorexia nervosa *is not a 'nervosa' or mental health problem* (Hay, 2021, p. 223). In her commentary on the findings which supported a conceptualisation of orthorexia nervosa as a positive state of being (He et al., 2021), Hay (2021) raises the question of whether orthorexia nervosa is a healthy way of being or is a mental health disorder. The author argues that in a mental health disorder, at the least, distress and/or dysfunction is required, such as in major diagnostic categories in the DSM-5 (Hay, 2021). Thus, orthorexia nervosa would be a mental health problem only when experienced by individuals with psychological distress and/ or interpersonal deficits. Thus, *orthorexia nervosa, as currently conceptualised, may not be a disorder in its own right but only when occurring in the context of another mental health or eating disorder* (Hay, 2021, pp. 223–224). In addition, the author emphasises that the Düsseldorf Orthorexia Scale appears to have not identified potentially pathological variants of orthorexic behaviour in the studied population (Hay, 2021). To better understand what state (healthy or unhealthy) orthorexia nervosa is, more empirical (experimental and longitudinal) studies with appropriate questionnaires, representative populations, and consideration of cultural relativity are required. The recent study (Li et al., 2022) conducted among two groups of college students in China ($N_1$ = 1289; 37.9%

women; $M_{age}$= 20.9±2.0 years and $N_2$ =1084; 68.1% women; $M_{age}$=21.0±2.3 years) found that male sex and satisfaction with weight and shape negatively predict orthorexia nervosa (assessed by the ORTO-R), whereas coffee drinking (at least once a week for six consecutive months), physical activities (exercising at least three times a week for at least 30 minutes each time), healthy food (consumption of legumes, dairy products and/or vegetables) and mental disorders (i.e. anxiety, depression or attention deficit and hyperactive disorder) are the factors positively associated with orthorexia nervosa. In addition, engagement in physical activities and the presence of mental disorders were related to orthorexia nervosa (assessed by ORTO-15) in Chinese college students.

## 12.2 South Korea

Epidemiological studies provide information about the distribution of disorders in a defined population and their trends over time (van Eeden, van Hoeken and Hoek, 2021). The previous study using a nationwide database (Lee et al., 2021) revealed that the treatment prevalence of eating disorders (with ICD F50.x) in South Korea was between 12.02 individuals per 100,000 (0.012%) in 2010 and 13.28 individuals per 100,000 (0.013%) in 2015. Regrettably, there is no population-representative epidemiological research on orthorexia nervosa in South Korea. In addition, there are only two studies investigating orthorexia nervosa in the Korean population.

At present, there is solely one case report (written in English) describing a male patient with orthorexia nervosa (Park et al., 2011). The patient ate only 3–4 spoons of brown rice and fresh vegetables without salt for three months, resulting in a 14 kg weight loss. He developed hyponatraemia (defined as a serum sodium level of less than 135 mEq/L; Adrogué et al., 2022), metabolic acidosis (characterised by an increase in the hydrogen ion concentration in the systemic circulation resulting in a serum HCO3 less than 24 mEq/L; Burger & Schaller, 2023), subcutaneous emphysema (the finding of air or gas beneath the skin; Melhorn & Davies, 2021), mediastinal emphysema (defines the presence of air in the mediastinum; Kouritas et al., 2015), pneumothorax (refers to air in the pleural cavity, i.e. interspersed between the lung and the chest wall; MacDuff et al., 2010) and pancytopenia (a decrease in all three blood cell lines and it could manifest with symptoms resulting from anaemia, leukopenia or thrombocytopenia; Gnanaraj et al., 2018). Only one existing study (Cho & Hyun, 2020), conducted among 321 adults (50.2% women; $M_{age}$ = 39.33±11.28 years), has demonstrated that 6.23% of the Korean women and men were classified as having orthorexia nervosa and 20.24% were at risk of developing orthorexia nervosa (assessed by the Düsseldorf Orthorexia Scale). In addition, weak negative associations were observed between orthorexia nervosa and the perceived severity of obesity and subjective evaluation of obesity degree (Cho & Hyun, 2020). These two variables had a significant negative effect on orthorexia nervosa. The relationships between orthorexia nervosa and sex, age, fear of obesity, body esteem and body satisfaction were not significant. The authors (Cho & Hyun, 2020) argue that orthorexia nervosa should be classified as an independent condition distinguished from anorexia nervosa.

## 12.3  Expert Commentary: Thoughts on Orthorexia Nervosa in Non-Western Societies

by Jinbo He, PhD

**Jinbo He**, PhD is Assistant Professor at the Chinese University of Hong Kong, Shenzhen. His primary research interests are eating behaviours and body image. He serves as the editorial board member for the International Journal of Eating Disorders, Body Image and Eating and Weight Disorders – Studies on Anorexia, Bulimia and Obesity.

Affiliation: Division of Applied Psychology, School of Humanities and Social Science, The Chinese University of Hong Kong, Shenzhen, China.

Orthorexia nervosa (ON) refers to pathological obsessions with healthy eating (Bratman & Knight, 2000). Since the emergence of this concept, ON has been mainly researched in Western societies, especially in Europe (Dunn & Bratman, 2016; Zhou et al., 2020). Only in recent years has ON been researched in non-Western societies, predominantly in Asian countries, such as Bangladesh (Sultana et al., 2022), China (He et al., 2019), India (Jain & Sharma, 2021), Iran (Eskandari et al., 2022), Lebanon (Haddad et al., 2020) and Turkey (Bağci Bosi, Camur & Güler, 2007; Taştekin Ouyaba & Çiçekoğlu Öztürk, 2022). However, compared to the fruitful findings of ON in Western societies, there is still very limited research evidence of ON in non-Western societies (Brytek-Matera et al., 2020). Thus, the present commentary aims to provide a brief commentary regarding ON in non-Western societies.

To date, available research about ON in non-Western societies is still very preliminary, as relevant studies are mostly in translation and are a validation of widely used instruments of ON, including the Düsseldorf Orthorexia Scale (DOS; Barthels, Meyer & Pietrowsky, 2015b) the Eating Habits Questionnaire (EHQ: Gleaves, Graham & Ambwani, 2013), the ORTO-15 (Donini et al.,

2005) and its refined version (i.e. ORTO-R; Rogoza & Donini, 2021) and the Teruel Orthorexia Scale (Barrada & Roncero, 2018). Except for the ORTO-15, which shows questionable psychometric properties, validation studies generally supported the use of these measures in specific non-Western countries, for example, the ORTO-R in China (Li et al., 2022), Lebanon (Rogoza et al., 2022) and Turkey (Özdengül et al., 2021), the DOS in China (He et al., 2019) and Lebanon (Rogoza et al., 2021; Hallit et al., 2021) and the EHQ (Hallit et al., 2021) and TOS (Mhanna et al., 2022) in Lebanon. However, it should be noted that perspectives on healthy eating differ by culture (Banna et al., 2016; Bisogni et al., 2012). For example, using a qualitative design, Banna and colleagues (2016) revealed several significant differences in perspectives on healthy eating between Chinese and American undergraduate students (e.g. Chinese undergraduate students emphasised regular timing of eating, while American undergraduate students emphasised balanced consumption of different food groups). Given that ON is tied to one's perceptions of healthy eating, it is important to further explore the unique manifestations of ON in non-Western societies by using measures developed in non-Western societies.

Furthermore, regarding the prevalence of ON in non-Western societies, most previous studies of ON used the ORTO-15 and reported extremely high prevalence rates (e.g. 75.2% in a representative sample of the Lebanese population; Haddad et al., 2019) However, due to the psychometric deficits in the ORTO-15 (Rogoza & Donini, 2021), the prevalence assessed by the ORTO-15 in non-Western countries might be inaccurate and overestimated. A sounder measurement of ON that can be used for screening purposes is the DOS (Barthels, Meyer & Pietrowsky, 2015b). The prevalence of ON, as measured by the DOS, was found to be 7.8% in a sample of Chinese undergraduate students and 19.5% in a sample of Chinese older adults (He et al., 2021). However, given that the DOS cannot differentiate orthorexia nervosa from healthy orthorexia (i.e. a non-pathological interest in healthy eating; Zickgraf & Barrada, 2022). In this regard, the prevalence based on the DOS might also be overestimated. In addition, even though the TOS distinguishes orthorexia nervosa and healthy orthorexia (Barrada & Roncero, 2018), no screening cut-offs have been developed for the TOS. Thus, the true prevalence of ON in non-Western countries remains unclear and should be re-examined in future studies with valid tools.

Finally, even though there have been studies in non-Western countries showing that ON is related to poorer well-being (e.g. higher disordered eating (Haddad et al., 2019), higher eating inflexibility (He et al., 2019), lower self-esteem (Yılmaz & Dundar, 2022), higher psychological distress (Yılmaz & Dundar, 2022; Zhou et al., 2020) and higher obsessive-compulsive symptoms (Zhou et al., 2020)), these prior studies were generally cross-sectional. In other words, longitudinal and experimental studies have still not tested the temporal and causal relationships between ON and any health correlates. Thus, further studies with longitudinal and experimental design studies are needed to identify the risk factors and health consequences of ON in non-Western societies.

# Highlights

- The research on orthorexia nervosa is most frequently based on convenience samples of students (e.g. Awad et al., 2022; Bundros et al., 2016; Brytek-Matera et al., 2020a; Cerolini et al., 2022; Costa & Hardan-Khalil, 2019) using the ORTO-15 and its modifications in most cases. Research findings into female predominance in orthorexia nervosa have been inconsistent and contradictory in both student samples and the general population. A great deal of previous research into orthorexia nervosa has focused on its relationship with other conditions. Vegetarianism and veganism appear to be associated with greater orthorexia nervosa pathology (see Brytek-Matera, 2021a; McLean, Kulkarni & Sharp, 2022), just like symptoms of eating disorder, obsessive-compulsive disorder and/or depression in both students and the general population (McComb & Mills, 2019). Additionally, several findings have identified the increased levels of anxiety and perfectionism associated with orthorexia nervosa in the general population. It has also been demonstrated that individuals with orthorexia nervosa were more likely to report higher levels of somatisation, maladaptive eating behaviour (e.g. restrained eating), stress, shame, health anxiety, negative affect, body image dissatisfaction and dysphoric body image emotions and lower levels of self-esteem and self-compassion. The longitudinal studies would help us to explain whether we could consider them the predisposing and/or maintaining factors of orthorexia nervosa.

- The evidence indicates that orthorexia nervosa is distinctively related to different psychopathological symptoms and conditions, which in turn suggests that orthorexia nervosa should be considered a condition with clinical significance rather than a lifestyle phenomenon (Håman et al., 2015). Despite existing limitations of the studies addressing convenience samples, the use of the criticised assessment tool (ORTO-15), cross-sectional design and little evidence classifying orthorexia nervosa as a mental illness (Strahler & Stark, 2020), we should remember that there are individuals with an abnormal preoccupation with healthy eating who experience difficulties in emotional, cognitive, behavioural and social everyday functioning. The research conducted among health professionals with clinical experience of individuals with orthorexia nervosa (e.g. Reynolds & McMahon, 2019; Sanzari & Hormes, 2023) and case reports (e.g. Lopes et al., 2020; Rania et al., 2021) provides evidence that orthorexia nervosa is undoubtedly an abnormal state of health.

Early intervention may potentially reduce the health impairment and improve the psychosocial functioning of patients with orthorexia nervosa. Therefore, there is a need to ensure appropriate treatment by qualified specialists.

• One longitudinal study of patients with eating disorders (Segura-Garcia et al., 2015) revealed an increased frequency of orthorexia nervosa after the treatment, in contrast to another study demonstrating that orthorexic tendencies are amenable to treatment for eating disorders (Hessler-Kaufmann et al., 2021). Orthorexia nervosa has been suggested to be independent of eating disorder pathology or represent less severe forms of eating disorders (Segura-Garcia et al., 2015). Moreover, orthorexia nervosa has been considered a coping strategy in patients with anorexia nervosa, representing a less pathological way to control food intake (Barthels et al., 2017). It has also been suggested that patients with eating disorders may perceive symptoms of orthorexia nervosa as adaptive and trend-informed eating styles that may serve as cover or legitimisation for a restrictive eating disorder (Hessler-Kaufmann et al., 2021). Orthorexia nervosa has also been proposed to be allocated to the eating disorder spectrum and likely represents a phenomenological subtype of a restrictive eating disorder rather than a distinct diagnosis (Hessler-Kaufmann et al., 2021). Other findings have highlighted the fact that orthorexia nervosa is strictly associated with the psychopathology of eating disorders (Brytek-Matera et al., 2015b; Busatta et al., 2022), which is not compatible with the assumption that patients with eating disorders may adopt orthorexic behaviours at the end of treatment as less unhealthy coping strategies to control food as well as body weight and shape (Barthels et al., 2017; Segura-Garcia et al., 2015). Moreover, the theory that orthorexia may be linked to a food-related acquaintance in patients with eating disorders (Barthels et al., 2017; Segura-Garcia et al., 2015) has not been confirmed in the recent study (Busatta et al., 2022). The assumptions that orthorexia nervosa is more prevalent among patients with obsessive-compulsive disorder than patients with other disorders (Poyraz et al., 2015) and healthy individuals (Yılmaz et al., 2020; Vaccari et al., 2021) have not been confirmed in the existing studies and there is no evidence for a relationship between orthorexia nervosa and obsessive-compulsive disorder in patients with obsessive-compulsive disorder (Yılmaz et al., 2020). Contrary to these findings, one clinical case (Rania et al., 2021) demonstrated that in a 32-year-old woman, obsessive-compulsive disorder preceded the onset of orthorexia nervosa. The inconsistency of the evidence leaves an important question open: whether clinicians ought to investigate the presence of the symptoms of orthorexia nervosa among patients with obsessive-compulsive disorder. Future longitudinal studies should investigate whether mental disorders and conditions contribute to the development of orthorexia nervosa in patients with a particular disease.

• Regarding non-Western societies, a recent study revealed that male students were more likely to have orthorexia nervosa in comparison to female students in Turkey (Yilmaz, 2023) and Jordan (Abdullah, Al Hourani & Alkhatib, 2020). While others have established that no significant sex differences in terms of orthorexia nervosa exist in the general population in Turkey (Kaya, Uzdil & Çakıroğlu, 2022; Sezer Katar, Şahin & Kurtoğlu, 2023). In addition, orthorexia nervosa was related to attitudes, feelings and behaviours related to eating pathology in the Turkish general population (Kaya, Uzdil & Çakıroğlu, 2022). In Lebanese adolescents, orthorexia nervosa was associated with higher levels of fearful-avoidant and preoccupied attachment styles, being female, and higher levels of physical activity, while higher levels of self-esteem were significantly linked to less orthorexic behaviours (Azzi et al., 2023). The typology of adolescents based on orthorexic eating behaviours has been proposed in a recent study (Yakın et al., 2022). Adolescents (aged between 15 and 18 years) in Lebanon with a moderate interest in healthy eating that has both pathological and healthy aspects (called 'moderate in-between orthorexia') had higher levels of anxiety, stress and depression and lower levels of self-esteem than those with no particular (healthy or pathological) interest in healthy eating (called 'low orthorexia'). Orthorexia nervosa was significantly weakly related to waterpipe smoking and unrelated to other lifestyle habits, namely cigarette smoking, alcohol consumption and physical activity among Lebanese adolescents (Samaha et al., 2022). Moreover, no significant relationship between orthorexia and age and sex was found in this group.

• The findings of the existing studies conducted among students in Mainland China have demonstrated that orthorexia nervosa is associated with higher levels of maladaptive eating behaviour (i.e. cognitive restraint, inflexible eating) (He et al., 2019), symptoms of different mental disorders or conditions (i.e. anxiety, depression, obsessive-compulsive disorder) (Li et al., 2022; Zhou et al., 2020) and fear of negative evaluation (Zhou et al., 2020). However, among women and men aged 51 to 92 years old, orthorexia nervosa was found to be associated with higher levels of positive body image and life satisfaction (He et al., 2021). All authors (He et al., 2019, 2021; Li et al., 2022; Zhou et al., 2020) emphasise the importance of investigating cultural specific as well as universal aspects of orthorexia nervosa in future research.

# Part VI

# Future Directions on Orthorexia Nervosa

# 13 Orthorexia Nervosa: What Do We Know and What Should We Do?

## 13.1 Expert Commentary: Musings on Orthorexia Nervosa

by Professor Phillipa Hay

**Phillipa Hay**, DPhil is Professor and Discipline Head of Mental Health at Western Sydney University and the Director of Mental Health Research for Mental Health Services at South Western Sydney Local Health District. Her major research interests are eating disorders, their treatment, phenomenology, distribution and determinants. Her research has been highly cited, award-winning and has included seminal papers, for example, in adapting care to peoples' preferences, the quality of life of people with eating disorders, and their presence in Indigenous peoples.

Affiliation: School of Medicine & Translational Health Research Institute, Western Sydney University, Sydney, Australia; and Mental Health Services, Camden and Campbelltown Hospitals, SWSLHD, Sydney, Australia.

Orthorexia nervosa is a syndrome not yet recognised in major classifications such as the DM-5 or ICD-11. At first glance, it may not even appear problematic. Its core feature is the pursuit of 'healthy' eating. In the same way as exercise has many positive attributes and psychological effects, and indeed can be regarded as a form of an antidepressant, desiring a nutritious diet may be promoted as a means of improving mood and well-being. The Royal Australian and New College of Psychiatrists (RANZCP) in their most recent Clinical Practice Guideline (Malhi et al., 2021) for management of mood disorders indeed have a section recommending dietary practices to enhance other treatments for low mood. They state that 'Diet with high proportions of vegetables, fruit, fish and grain but low animal fats appear helpful in depressive disorders' (p. 38).

However, it does appear that sometimes the desire to be healthy is taken to an extreme. How may this then become a disorder? The Diagnostic and Statistical Manual of Mental Disorders, Fifth edition (DSM-5; APA, 2013) requires distress and/or impact on daily function to elevate problematic behavioural from the sphere of normal experience to mental ill health. Thus, a diet that reduces the person's ability to eat with others, to engage in social activities around food, and where there is distress if the person cannot keep to their self-imposed diet (e.g. when selected foods become unavailable) can be argued to reach diagnostic criteria. One would expect that this scenario would include distracting preoccupations about food and eating and emotions of dysphoria and anxiety around food accessibility, such as are found in people with eating disorders. That the behaviours are not driven by a desire to lose weight is no longer a reason to exclude orthorexia nervosa from the eating disorders group as this is not a criteria for other recognised feeding and eating disorders such a avoidant/restrictive food intake disorder (ARFID) or binge eating disorder. In this regard an international consortium has proposed criteria that include consequences as well as core features of orthorexia nervosa (Donini et al., 2022).

It is important to consider the consequences of orthorexia nervosa symptoms as not all people with these become distressed or experience extreme preoccupations and impacts on their daily life. Early research papers used a broad insument not well-designed to identify this, that is, the ORTHO-15 test (Donini et al., 2004). Studies using this tool often reported a very high prevalence of orthorexia nervosa behaviours in community samples of tertiary students or others (e.g. Brytek-Matera et al., 2015a, 2016). On the one hand, it could be surmised that these behaviours are part of the normal experience of living in an environment where both food is replete and where public health concerns about the quality and quantity of consumption are high.

On the other hand, these studies (e.g. Brytek-Matera et al., 2015a, 2016) have found associations between orthorexia nervosa behaviours and symptoms of eating disorders. In the same way that restrictive dieting to improve health and weight is an acceptable and common behaviour, but anorexia nervosa is an illness, so may be orthorexia nervosa. It is only where it becomes extreme and impacts on the person's psychosocial function and their physical and mental health that a diagnosis is made. Applying such parameters reduces the estimated prevalence of orthorexia nervosa to around 1% (Dunn et al., 2017), and its inclusion in the DSM would be supported.

However, may orthorexia nervosa impact on people's health in a positive direction? A paper that I have previously commented on (Hay, 2020) found positive impacts on quality of life and well-being and body dissatisfaction for older people from China who were engaging in orthorexia nervosa behaviours (He at al., 2021). This study also used one of the more recent validated assessment tools to identify orthorexia nervosa, that is, the Düsseldorf Orthorexia Scale (C-DOS; He, et al., 2019). It was challenging to know what to make of the findings. Perhaps, orthorexia nervosa should be regarded as a disorder that may be, to a degree, located in culture and time. Are we imposing cultural attitudes and beliefs on behaviours and generating distress and illness?

A case in point is the twentieth-century aberration whereby normative love between people of the same gender became a disorder. It led to the exile and likely early death of one of the most gifted writers in the English-speaking world, Oscar Wilde. In his novel Maurice, Forster (himself a gay person; Hastings, 2012; Nadel, 1982) wrote of the ridiculous attempts to treat the protagonist and cure him. It is salutary to note that it was only in 1973 that homosexuality was written out of the DSM (Drescher, 2015). It is likely easier to create a disorder than to lose one as the increasing size of the DSM and Mental Health chapter of the ICD attest to. And was it so inappropriate? People who identified as homosexual in the mid twentieth century in the English-speaking world could be forgiven for thinking that there was something fundamentally wrong with them. They likely had recurrent distressing preoccupations about their sexuality and self-doubt. With encouragement from psychiatrists and, if unlucky, directives from courts of law, they would have taken agents harmful to their physical and emotional health to supress their sexuality. The 2014 film The Imitation Game poignantly evoked the life-threatening impacts of such treatments for one of the century's greatest scientists, Alan Turing.

Am I drawing 'too long a bow'? In my personal clinical experience, I have met few individuals with orthorexia nervosa. Prior to the DSM-5, when people have presented with food restriction to the point that it has impacted on their physical and/or mental health but without a drive to lose weight or other body image concerns, I would have made the diagnosis of atypical anorexia nervosa, and since the DSM-5, the diagnosis of ARFID. However, the lack of help-seeking or large presence in eating disorder clinics is not a reason to dismiss orthorexia nervosa as a disorder. The situation was very similar up to very recently for people with binge eating disorder. Some people do seek help and have developed physical and mental health sequelae of orthorexia behaviours and related quality of life impairments. Unlike homosexuality, orthorexia nervosa is not innate. Innate traits such as a high level of asceticism as in the nursery rhyme 'Jack Spratt' who could eat no fat, or traits that also predispose to anorexic nervosa such as clinical perfectionism (McComb & Mills, 2019), may increase a person's risk for orthorexia nervosa. But orthorexia nervosa is not inborn and people can recover from it and live more fulfilling lives as a result (McGovern, Gaffney Trimble, 2021).

Thus, on balance, I'm of the view that orthorexia nervosa will be recognised as an eating disorder, or a variant of an eating disorder such as ARFID, and we will see more people in need of help. This may take the form of modifying behaviours and extreme beliefs and enabling the person to develop an identity and positive self-regard independent of the disorder. To inform the development of treatments and further refine phenomenology, research is needed to explore the lived experience of people with high levels of orthorexia nervosa symptoms. This needs to be in non-clinical settings, before the selection bias of engaging with healthcare systems occurs. The present book is a timely initiative to help drive the field forward in understanding the phenomenology of orthorexia nervosa and also its assessment and treatment.

## 13.2  Eating Healthily: Health Promotive Perspective

Several factors, including intra-individual factors (such as physiological and psychological factors, acquired food preferences and knowledge), interpersonal or social factors (such as family and group influences), and cultural and economic factors, contribute to the development, maintenance and change of dietary patterns (Eertmans, Baeyens & Van den Bergh, 2001). Eertmans, Baeyens Van den Bergh (2001) developed a hypothetical food choice and intake model, presenting various determinants influencing eating behaviour (Figure 13.1). The model includes three levels of variables and their interrelationships. Food-internal (e.g. flavour) and food-external (e.g. information on healthy food aspects, the social environment and the physical environment) stimuli are located on the first or independent level. Information about healthy food aspects sometimes emerges to have a positive effect on liking, sometimes a negative effect and sometimes no effect at all. Also, information-based expectations can affect high or low food liking. Other important moderating factors in the association between information and food liking are individuals' attitudes towards nutrition or their concern for the health consequences of ingesting specific foods. Social factors seem to influence eating behaviour through social facilitation (resulting in increased food intake when eating in the presence of others, through establishing family food rules at a younger age

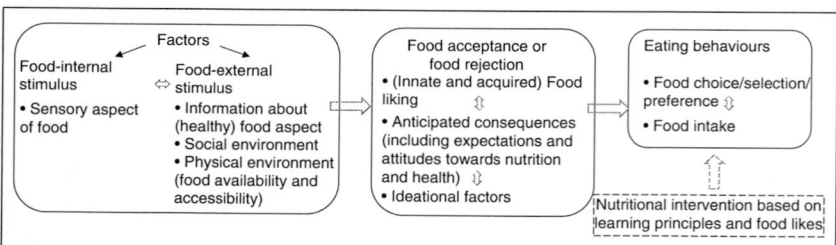

Figure 13.1  Hypothetical model presenting various determinants influencing eating behaviour.
Source: Based on Eertmans, Baeyens & Van den Bergh (2001).

or through various learning mechanisms). The food taxonomy is located on the second or the intermediate level. It categorises food acceptance or rejection criteria: food liking (innate and acquired), anticipated consequences (including expectations and attitudes towards nutrition and health) and ideational factors. Liking, or the affective response to a food's sensory properties, is considered the best predictor of food choice or intake in the absence of economic and availability constraints and appears to be at the centre of the development, maintenance and change of dietary patterns. Regarding acquired food likes, processes of mere exposure, Pavlovian conditioning (which may be the principal process in acquiring food (dis)likes) and social learning are relevant learning mechanisms involved in eating behaviour that shape associations between liking and other determinants. Finally, eating behaviour is regarded as the ultimate dependent variable, operationalised either as food choice/selection/preference or as food intake. Both the food taxonomy and eating behaviour are dependent on food-internal and food-external stimuli (Eertmans, Baeyens & Van den Bergh, 2001).

Efforts to promote healthy eating behaviour might benefit from increased attention towards learning principles and food preferences in the design of interventions. Experience with the food should include experience with its taste and not merely its visual aspects. If liking is that relevant a determinant of food choice, health professionals should focus their efforts on processes determining liking to improve food choice (Eertmans, Baeyens & Van den Bergh, 2001).

Over 100 countries have developed food-based dietary guidelines (FAO, 2015). They have been described as science-based recommendations in the form of guidelines for healthy eating (European Food Safety Authority, 2010). In European countries, food groupings and food group names differ across individual food-based dietary guidelines. However, the number of portions and portion sizes are kept unaltered. A key feature of the food-based dietary guidelines is that they focus on desirable dietary patterns, not specific nutrients (Green, 2015). The UK government's healthy eating recommendations are visually depicted in the Eatwell Guide (see Section 1.1, Figure 1.1 in Chapter 1), one of the many examples of a healthy eating tool that uses food-based dietary guidelines (Green, 2015). In parallel with food-based dietary guidelines, there is authoritative dietary advice about single nutrients, especially those of public health relevance (e.g. lower free sugar consumption) (Green, 2015).

In promoting healthy nutrition, dietary recommendations should focus on *what* and *how* to eat for optimal health, healthy eating behaviours and food acceptance. Dietary guidelines should focus on those components (foods and nutrients) that characterise healthful diets (Green, 2015). Food-based dietary recommendations founded on different dietary patterns (e.g. Mediterranean-style, a healthy vegetarian diet) help to facilitate personal preferences (e.g. taste, cost, convenience, culture) for different foods (Green, 2015). Individuals looking for dietary guidance can find food-based dietary guidelines (e.g. Eatwell Guide) and recommended nutrient intakes (e.g. nutrition labelling on packaged foods). A range of communication approaches are needed to help individuals eat healthfully, including nutrition labelling and information about serving size and frequency of consumption (Green, 2015). Recently, FABLE – Food and Beverages Labels Explorer, a web-based Europe-wide nutrition information tool (www.food-labels-explorer.jrc.ec.europa.eu/en) containing general and nutritional information from the labels of packaged foods and beverages in Europe, has been proposed to monitor the nutritional quality of the food (European Commission, 2023). Sufficient knowledge and understanding of nutrition would help choose a healthful diet. However, we should consider that nutritional needs vary according to sex, life stage, lifestyle and health status. In addition, the impact of nutrients on biomarkers for health is influenced by an individual's genetic background (Green, 2015). Repeated exposure to new foods is an effective strategy to increase the acceptability of foods and their intake in adults (Eertmans, Baeyens & Van den Bergh, 2001). Having positive experiences by consuming diverse foods may influence their acceptance and foster individuals to make expanded food choices and healthy eating decisions. Positive strategies that recognise the importance of eating pleasure may effectively change perceptions about healthy eating (Vaillancourt et al., 2019). Considering that affective messages were found to be more effective than cognitive messages in favouring behavioural changes, efforts to promote healthy eating that target affective attitudes, such as a pleasure-oriented approach, could be more powerful at fostering dietary behaviour changes than efforts appealing solely to cognitive outcomes and functional considerations of food such as the health-oriented approach. However, additional intervention studies are needed to confirm this hypothesis (Vaillancourt et al., 2019). Beliefs and knowledge regarding a particular product are thought to positively affect food preference and its acceptability (Simons & Hall, 2017). Although sustaining healthy behaviours is difficult, guided, individualised counselling and support from a nutritional professional may facilitate the process of achieving sustainable changes in individuals' eating patterns (Mattei & Alfonso, 2020). Health promotion interventions, such as health education and nutrition education, could also help maintain a healthy eating pattern.

## 13.3  Holistic Approach to Orthorexia Nervosa Treatment

At present, there is an apparent lack of coherent conceptualisation of orthorexia nervosa. Recently, orthorexia nervosa has been conceptualised in the context of eating disorders, a safety mechanism for health anxieties, health perfectionism, the pursuit of superiority, as well as obsessive practice and response to anxiety to differentiate it from self-chosen dietary ideals (Opitz, Newman & Sharpe, 2022). Depending on the conceptualisation of orthorexia nervosa, the appropriate treatment would be recommended. Classifying orthorexia nervosa under the current diagnostic criteria of anorexia nervosa (Bhattacharya et al., 2022) may permit us to use the enhanced form of cognitive behavioural therapy (CBT-E) in the treatment of patients with orthorexia nervosa. The CBT-E has been used to treat outpatients with anorexia nervosa, with a good outcome in approximately 60% of them and a low relapse rate (Fairburn, 2009 in Murphy et al., 2010). CBT-E has been scientifically supported to be effective in the treatment of both adults (Fairburn et al., 2013) and adolescents with eating disorders (Dalle Grave et al., 2013). It is recommended by the National Institute for Health and Care Excellence (NICE, 2017). CBT-E has been found to promote weight restoration to a healthy weight (Calugi et al., 2015) and decrease eating disorder symptoms (Kessler et al., 2022). Other evidence-based therapies for anorexia nervosa are the Maudsley Anorexia Nervosa Therapy for Adults and Specialist Supportive Clinical Management (Table 13.1). They provide psychoeducation and aim to restore the individual's physical health with weight monitoring, nutritional counselling and meal planning, often alongside sessions from a registered dietitian (Hay, 2020).

In the case of conceptualisation of orthorexia nervosa as a manifestation of obsessive-compulsive disorder, with intrusive thoughts about health and food being managed through avoidance and ritualising, which are negatively reinforced by temporary relief from anxiety, the method of exposure and response prevention, which is considered to be the first line treatment for obsessive-compulsive disorder (Nezgovorova et al., 2022), is recommended to help patients recognise and interrupt the cycle of anxiety and avoidance (Zickgraf, 2020). Exposure and response prevention focuses on eliminating rituals and avoidance behaviours and teaching patients to tolerate distress without engaging in counterproductive behaviours (Hezel & Simpson, 2019). Exposure and response prevention are divided into several stages: (1) identification of external (e.g. situations, objects, people) and internal (thoughts and physiological reactions) stimuli that trigger the patient's obsessive thoughts and subsequent distress; (2) identification of the specific content of the patient's obsessions and

Table 13.1 Conceptualisation of orthorexia nervosa in relation to anorexia nervosa: consideration regarding the treatment of orthorexia nervosa

Effective treatments of anorexia nervosa aimed at improving its symptoms and restoring weight

Cognitive behavioural therapy (CBT) and Cognitive Behaviour Therapy – Enhanced (CBT-E)

- The activities of directly challenging anorexia-related behaviours, dysfunctional beliefs (cognitions and patterns of thinking), especially symptoms maintaining anorexia nervosa.
- Cognitive restructuring, behavioural monitoring, behavioural experiments and chain analyses are the techniques used in CBT and CBT-E.

Specialist supportive clinical management (SSCM)

- The resumption of normal eating and the restoration of weight; a flexible approach to addressing life issues impacting anorexia nervosa.
- Psychoeducation and supportive therapy are used in SSCM.

The Maudsley Model of Anorexia Nervosa Treatment For Adults (MANTRA)

- Addressing the obsessional and anxious/avoidant traits that are proposed as being central to the maintenance of anorexia nervosa.
- MANTRA draws on a range of approaches, including motivational interviewing, cognitive remediation and social integration (e.g. flexible involvement of carers).

Motivation-based therapies (e.g. motivational interviewing, motivational enhancement), either as the main therapy or in conjunction with another therapy

- Improving an individual's motivation and engagement to change.
- Use of the techniques to enhance change.

Family therapies and a specific form of family therapy are termed 'family-based treatment'

- The involvement of family in treatment.

Source: Based on Hay et al. (2014) and Hay (2020).

compulsions, discussion of the functional relationship between the two, and identification of the feared outcome if the rituals are not performed; (3) ranking of different situations in order from least to most distressing (as measured by subjective units of distress), which results in a fear hierarchy; (4) making the patient aware that she or he repeatedly confronts the situations on her or his fear hierarchy while refraining from engaging in compulsions. By practising both in vivo and imaginal exposures, the patient learns that the consequences of her or his fear do not occur, as well as how to tolerate distress and uncertainty without engaging in compulsions; (5) following each in-session exposure, engagement of the patient in post-exposure processing to review her or his experience and how her or his expectations were violated and what she or he learned; (6) as patient habituates to various scenarios, she or he then gradually work her or his way up the fear hierarchy to confront increasingly distressing situations; (7) a course of exposure and response prevention concludes with relapse prevention planning (Hezel & Simpson, 2019).

There is currently not enough reliable evidence to describe the appropriate treatment of orthorexia nervosa due to an insufficient number of studies on treatment recommendations (Horovitz & Argyrides, 2023; Koven & Abry, 2015; Zickgraf, 2020). Moreover, there is no research focusing on treatment effectiveness, as well as no evidence-based treatment for orthorexia nervosa (Brytek-Matera, 2023; Zickgraf, 2020). However, some suggestions for the treatment of this phenomenon have been previously proposed (Koven & Abry, 2015): a multidisciplinary team approach (including physicians, psychotherapists and dieticians), the use of psychoeducation on nutrition and health (for minimalising false food and health beliefs), the use of cognitive restructuring (beneficial, e.g. dichotomous thinking, overgeneralisation, and other cognitive distortions surrounding food, eating and health) and behaviour modification strategies (e.g. for increasing socialisation during meals) as well as exposure and response prevention potentially in conjunction with habit reversal training. A combination of cognitive behavioural therapy, psychoeducation and medication has been proposed as an effective treatment for orthorexia nervosa (Koven & Abry, 2015). Cognitive behavioural therapy, oriented on maladaptive thought processes and behaviours resulting from the occurrence of orthorexia nervosa, would allow patients to learn to identify and reframe rigid and unhealthy thoughts about food, healthy eating and health and regulate negative emotions that frequently occur as a result of dietary deviations, whereas psychoeducation would help the patients assess their attitude towards orthorexia nervosa. Psychoeducation facilitates patients' understanding of their behaviours and helps them change their thinking. However, it should not be as considered an alternative form of therapy, as its aim is not to modify the beliefs and thinking causing certain behaviours. To be effective, it needs to be incorporated into cognitive and behavioural strategies that enable the patient to verify new information (Waller et al., 2007). Suggestions for key topics worth including in a psychoeducation programme with individuals with orthorexia nervosa are presented in Table 13.2.

Although no reported studies are exploring the use of psychotropic medications in patients with orthorexia nervosa, serotonin reuptake inhibitors have been considered beneficial for patients with orthorexia nervosa with

Table 13.2 Key topics of psychoeducation within intervention with individuals with orthorexia nervosa

| *Key topics* |
|---|
| • Recommendations of dietary energy intake for the attainment and maintenance of optimal health, physiological function and well-being |
| • Objective healthy diet[a] (see Chapter 1) versus subjective healthy diet[b] |
| • Health behaviours (see Section 2.1 in Chapter 2): health-enhancing behaviour versus health-impairing behaviour (e.g. see Table 2.1) |
| • Psychological, social and medical consequences of the limited food choices |

Note: [a] An adequate, healthy diet must satisfy human needs for energy and all essential nutrients (WHO, 2018, 2020); Eatwell Guide (see Figure 1.1 in Chapter 1); [b] Omission of certain foods or entire food groups believed to be unhealthy or impure; 'selectivity' of food.

anxiety and obsessive-compulsive traits (Mathieu, 2005). Nevertheless, the use of medications can be refused by these patients because of their unnatural composition (Mathieu, 2005).

Nutritional counselling (for restoring a healthy and balanced relationship with food), intuitive eating approaches (for overcoming rigid dietary rules and adopting a more mindful and non-judgmental approach to eating, promoting self-compassion and body acceptance) and mindfulness and acceptance-based treatment (for providing a healthy relationship with food and psychological well-being) have been proposed as promising methods in the comprehensive treatment of orthorexia nervosa (Horovitz & Argyrides, 2023).

Until now, only one qualitative study (McGovern, Gaffney & Trimble, 2021) has presented the experience of orthorexia nervosa from the perspective of recovered individuals who had been diagnosed with orthorexia nervosa by a health professional or had formerly met the criteria proposed by Dunn and Bratman (2016). In these individuals who no longer met the criteria for orthorexia nervosa for at least one year ($N = 8$), orthorexia nervosa began as a diet or as an interest in nutrition. Orthorexia nervosa had a critical impact on their emotional and social life. It contributed to obsession with diet, negative emotional states (e.g. anxiety about food choices), as well as social isolation and negative interpersonal relationships (family, partner and friend relationships). These individuals had experienced an eating disorder before developing orthorexia nervosa or during orthorexia nervosa as well, and they had experienced compensatory behaviours (e.g. binge eating with and without purging, fasting and meal skipping). Most individuals had concerns over weight and body image and reported both physical (e.g. insomnia, gastrointestinal distress) and mental health difficulties (McGovern, Gaffney & Trimble, 2021). Similar experiences were found among individuals self-diagnosed with (Valente et al., 2020) or self-identified (Talbot, Campbell & Greville-Harris, 2023) orthorexia nervosa. Concerns about health, interpersonal difficulties and the desire to find freedom from food rules and to establish a healthy relationship with food (Talbot, Campbell & Greville-Harris, 2023) may enhance a perception of a need for treatment in individuals with orthorexia nervosa. Previous research has established that individuals with higher levels of orthorexic symptomology and eating disorder symptomology, as well as those who recognise their healthy eating as problematic, are significantly more likely to have a perceived need for treatment (Walker-Swanton, Hay & Conti, 2020). Individuals with orthorexia nervosa may be prone to treatment due to their concern for their health (Brytek-Matera, 2012). Help-seeking addresses a health concern and does not result from eating behaviours they perceive as normative and healthy. Perhaps viewing treatment-seeking as ego-syntonic and a way of improving health and wellness together with more significant health literacy (Walker-Swanton, Hay & Conti, 2020) makes them willing to undergo treatment. It cannot be ruled out that the presence of emotional distress also contributes to seeking help from health professionals.

To sum up, research and discussion are urgently needed on the treatment of orthorexia nervosa to know how orthorexia nervosa should be treated (similarly to anorexia nervosa or obsessive-compulsive disorders or another condition) and which specific therapy/interventions work(s) best for these individuals.

## How Can Specialists Assess Orthorexia Nervosa?

The clinical assessment of the patient is the collecting of information and concluding the use of observation (e.g. naturalistic or laboratory), psychological tests, neurological tests and clinical interviews (unstructured or semi-structured or structured) (Bridley & Daffin, 2023). Guidelines developed for the assessment of eating disorders and related symptomatology (Anderson et al., 2018) may be considered for use in the assessment of orthorexia nervosa. The assessment process starts with broad considerations about the context in which the assessment is to be given, and the assessment process ends with the choice of specific instruments (Anderson et al., 2018). It is composed of four steps with a key question in each: the context of the assessment ('where'), the function of the assessment ('why'), the constructs of interest ('what'), and the specific instruments in the assessment ('how') (Figure 13.2).

In the first step, the function of an assessment is the 'where' of the assessment process. There is a need to determine under what circumstances the

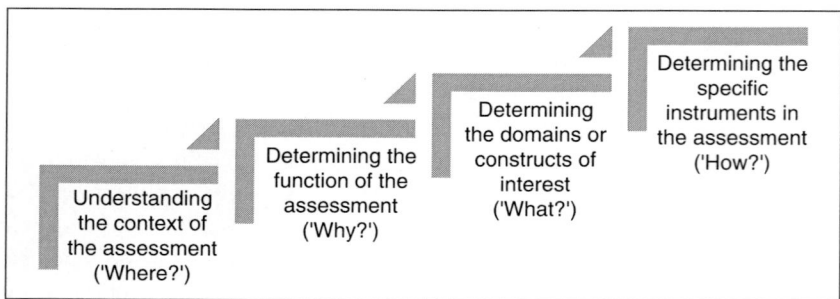

**Figure 13.2** The assessment process: steps and key questions used in the assessment of eating disorders and eating-related problems.
*Source*: Based on Anderson et al. (2018).

assessment occurs (e.g. in an inpatient psychiatric treatment facility or at an outpatient treatment session). The notion of context is intimately connected with the function of the assessment (the second step). The function of the assessment is the 'why' of the assessment process. There is a need to determine why exactly the assessment is being conducted. The potential functions for an assessment can be grouped into a few common categories that can overlap: screening (see as a proposal Orthorexia Nervosa Screening Questions in Table 6.7 in Chapter 6), diagnosis (see Chapter 4), treatment planning (see Section 13.2) and treatment outcome (that refers to 'changes in condition (psychological, somatic, physical, social and cultural) reflecting favourable or adverse impacts on the patient well-being'; Orlinski, Grawe & Parks, 1994, p. 284). Determining the exact domains or constructs relevant to the assessment question is the third step in the assessment process. The domains or constructs of the assessment are the 'what' of the assessment process. There is a need to determine what specific attitudes, thoughts and behaviours should be assessed. In the fourth step, the specific instruments in the assessment are the 'how' of the assessment process. There is a need to determine how the domains identified in the previous step should be assessed (e.g. using interviews, self-report questionnaires for screening, diagnosis and treatment planning and evaluation, as well as self-monitoring particularly useful for tracking treatment progress) (Anderson et al., 2018).

Currently, specialists are unable to 'diagnose' orthorexia nervosa in a standardised way. The current state of knowledge and research allows them to use the recent diagnostic criteria (proposed by Dunn & Bratman, 2016) and the measures that appear reliable to measure orthorexia nervosa symptomatology (e.g. the Eating Habits Questionnaire and the Düsseldorf Orthorexia Scale).

## 13.4 Expert Commentary: Thoughts on Orthorexia Nervosa – Past, Present and Future Perspectives

by Professor Thom Dunn

**Thom Dunn**, PhD is Professor of Psychological Sciences at the University of Northern Colorado and part of the Behavioral Health faculty at Denver Health. His major research interests are eating disorders that lead to malnutrition without disrupted body image. He was the 2021 recipient of a local humanitarian award by early career psychologists.

Affiliation: University of Northern Colorado, Greeley, United States of America.

As a clinical psychologist in academia, I routinely balance my clinical duties with research ones. I was therefore fascinated in 2014 to meet a young man who presented to my hospital after a 30 kg weight loss and malnourishment. I was struck, at the time, by what I perceived to be a man who was psychotic and delusional about his need for micronutrients. Further, his low body weight and associated medical complications were entirely about the purity of his diet. 'They tell me that I have orthorexia nervosa,' he said. 'But I just want to be healthy.' I had never heard of the term.

I worked with a resident physician on writing up the case, our article being the first that had been published in a widely distributed US psychiatry journal (Moroze et al., 2015). Shortly after this article was released, a social media figure Jordan Younger (aka 'The Blonde Vegan'), posted about her struggle with being too healthy in her diet, announcing she was living with orthorexia nervosa (ON). This provoked considerable media attention and when reporters and editors were looking to experts in the area, our paper was new and we were inundated with media requests. The need for additional work in the area of pathologically healthful eating was quite apparent and I shifted my research focus to ON.

There is no doubt that among the most important events in advancing the study of ON was the early work of Lorenzo Donini and his colleagues in Italy, with peer-reviewed publications (Donini et al., 2004, 2005) appearing only a few years after Bratman's book was published (Bratman & Knight, 2000). This was pivotal, as it elevated the discussion of pathologically healthful eating from the lay press to the professional one. This then spurred a flurry of publications, most of them using the 'ORTO-15', or a derivative, as a measure of ON. These early efforts were equally important, as they continued the discourse of ON in the eating disorder literature. However, as later authors have written

(Dunn & Bratman, 2016; Dunn et al., 2017; Heiss et al., 2019; Missbach et al., 2015; Mitrofanova et al., 2021), the ORTO-15 (and its derivatives) have poor psychometric properties and are likely detecting non-pathologically healthful eating rather than ON. This, unfortunately, as led to dozens of thoughtful papers drawing conclusions about ON and its nature that have unfortunately been based on data from the ORTO-15 family. Great scepticism should be exercised with any work using such instruments, as they misidentify those with healthy eating as those living with ON.

In the two decades that have passed since Bratman's book was published, I fear that the field of ON is still fledgling, largely because there seems to be a chasm between those who treat ON and those who research it. In my review of the literature, there is a poverty of studies of samples of individuals who are living with ON, and who have been diagnosed using one of the prominent diagnostic criteria sets. Instead, the literature is dominated by studies of individuals from convenience samples, predominantly university students. A great deal of these studies are correlational in nature, looking to identify trends associated with instruments purportedly identifying ON. Rarely, though, do these studies use diagnostic criteria sets to first identify those likely living with ON, and then examine this subgroup, which would be a stronger experimental design.

As we move into the third decade of research and discussion of ON, I believe there are several salient points that are important to make:

First – while other authors have written about various types of disordered eating, such as 'Bigorexia' or 'Drunkorexia', these have not generated the same attention as ON. For example, Google lists more than million hits when searching on 'Orthorexia', while Bigorexia has just more than 100,000. I suspect that is because ON is far more prevalent. It is also clear that ON is not a 'fad' as some have wondered (Vandereycken, 2011).

Second – still, twenty years after it first started being discussed, there is ongoing issues of clarity about diagnosing ON, as there is no codified diagnosis in major classification systems, such as inclusion in either the International Classification of Disease or the Diagnostic and Statistical Manual of Mental Disorders. I was one of many who looked to make an argument to the American Psychiatric Association that ON should be considered for inclusion in the latest revision of the DSM. Their criteria for an addition of a disorder are quite high and the scientific inquiry is still insufficient. I agree with others (Meule & Voderholzer, 2022) when I suspect that those interested in ON will be best served by looking to modify criteria of an existing condition. I argue for reconsidering the concept of restrictive eating leading to weight loss being so closely tied to body image.

Third – I believe that we need to be very cautious suggesting that there is such a thing as 'healthy' or 'non-pathological' ON (Yakin, Raynal & Chabrol, 2022; Zickgraf & Barrada, 2021). The concept of pathologically healthful eating comes under attack from individuals who believe its proponents are anti-health. Ross Arguedas (2020), for example, writes that the diagnosis of ON 'invites a re-interpretation of healthy dieting practices'. A literature of 'healthy orthorexia' gives fodder for these critics and does little to advance the understanding of the topic. There is no such thing as 'healthy anorexia', for example, and suggesting so is absurd. Instead, I believe these scholars really mean 'subclinical' ON. That is, somewhat extreme healthful eating that does not lead to malnutrition, nor other daily impairment. This is important to study because I have the sense (anecdotally) that it is prevalent and we need a broader understanding of how this represents disordered eating that may become pathological.

Fourth – people die from ON. I believe its most insidious form is when people start using 'food as medicine'. That is, there are some who get so carried away about adjusting their diet to cope with a medical condition that they become quite malnourished (Park et al., 2011). Indeed, I personally treated a 60-year-old man whose rigid diet of healthy heating 'prescribed' by his chiropractor led to severe restriction of his diet, ultimately leading to his death. Assessing beliefs of food as medicine is critical.

I am optimistic about the growing literature of ON and increasing its understanding. It is imperative; lives depend on it.

## 13.5 Future Research Directions

*Only to the extent we are able to explain empirical facts can we obtain the major objective of scientific research, namely not merely to record the phenomena of our experience, but to learn from them, by basing upon them theoretical generalizations which enable us to anticipate new occurrences and to control, at least to some extent, the changes in our environment* (Brody, 1970 in Kukull & Ganguli, 2012).

Thus far, there are conceptual and methodological issues associated with orthorexia nervosa. Despite the intensive research conducted in recent years in the area of orthorexia nervosa, no consensus on the definition has been reached. The definition of orthorexia nervosa should have been updated (Thorsberg, 2022; see Section 3.1.1 in Chapter 3); therefore, a conceptual review is needed to propose a new definition. The current state of research does not allow the final categorisation of orthorexia nervosa as a distinct diagnostic category (Cuzzolaro & Donini, 2016). Thus, more empirical evidence is required to attempt to explain what kind of condition orthorexia nervosa is and to clarify whether this phenomenon should be considered a separate nosological entity (Hessler-Kaufmann et al., 2021) or a new eating disorder (Cosh et al., 2023) or whether orthorexia nervosa instead falls under the umbrella of anorexia nervosa (Bhattacharya et al., 2022) or whether we might classify the severe and pathological manifestations of orthorexia nervosa (with clinical and functional impact) as another specified feeding or eating disorder or unspecified feeding or eating disorder for the moment, as it is not possible to consider it as a valid and specific category (Brytek-Matera, 2023). However, several propositions for the diagnosis of orthorexia nervosa (see Chapter 4) still lack the standardised diagnostic criteria. Validated diagnostic criteria for orthorexia nervosa would help advance clinical and research efforts into its prevalence, risk factors, therapeutic intervention and treatment. Differentiation between extremely healthy eating behaviour causing health problems and health protection by a healthy diet (Bóna, Túry & Forgácsc, 2019) should also be considered in the foreseeable future. In other words, it is necessary to distinguish orthorexia nervosa from normative eating behaviours that promote healthy lifestyle behaviours and help individuals attain personal goals related to health (Brytek-Matera, 2023).

Due to the critical views on the ORTO-15 as an unreliable and invalid measure of orthorexia nervosa, and consequently, postulation of discontinued use of this tool to assess orthorexia nervosa (e.g. Opitz et al., 2020; Meule et al., 2020; Missbach et al., 2017) the results obtained from the ORTO-15 should be interpreted with caution (Niedzielski & Kazmierczak-Wojtaś, 2021). There is also the question of whether these findings should be listed in the systematic reviews and meta-analyses. The use of an unreliable measure constitutes a threat to our understanding of orthorexia nervosa. We can only confirm the findings if the measurement is reliable (Rodebaugh et al., 2016). Therefore, the use of other questionnaires evaluating orthorexia nervosa has been suggested (see Part III). Although several different tools are available, there is no universal one best suited to measure the diagnosis of orthorexia nervosa. This points towards a topic to be addressed in future research.

Our current knowledge of orthorexia nervosa is not based on clinical case reports, observational studies or longitudinal studies but predominantly on cross-sectional studies. Choosing a cross-sectional research design helps describe the current state of orthorexia nervosa, identify associations between orthorexia nervosa and other variables, and compare different (non-clinical and clinical) groups. However, a cross-sectional design is inappropriate for establishing causal relationships, tracking changes over time, and evaluating effects (what longitudinal research allows) (Table 13.3).

Research on orthorexia nervosa in college and/or university students is rapidly increasing. Unfortunately, these studies inhibit the generalisability of

**Table 13.3** Strengths, weaknesses and reporting considerations of the cross-sectional studies

Benefits

- Relatively quick and inexpensive to conduct
- Determination of the prevalence
- Investigation of the relationship between multiple exposures and outcomes
- In most cases, using self-reported questionnaires or interviews
- Data collection at a one-time point
- Possibility of studying the multiple outcomes and exposures
- Possibility of creating an in-depth research study using the cross-cultural findings

Downsides

- Using questionnaires to reach a large sample of the population of interest can result in low response rates
- The inability to measure the incidence
- The inability to make a causal inference
- The inability to investigate the temporal relation between outcomes and risk factors
- Susceptible to sampling bias (e.g. non-response bias, recall bias)

Recommendations

- The full and transparent reporting of information on all aspects of a cross-sectional study by following the Strengthening the Reporting of Observational Studies in Epidemiology (STROBE) statement or the Transparent Reporting of a Multivariable Prediction Model for Individual Prognosis or Diagnosis (TRIPOD) statement (in the case of development of the diagnostic prediction models). Both contain a checklist of 22 items that are considered essential to report.

*Source*: Based on Wang and Cheng (2020).

results to the larger population, which is associated with certain limitations. The dearth of sample diversity in research on orthorexia nervosa (Valente et al., 2019) directly affects the validity and reliability of research findings and results in more inaccurate generalisations (Hall, 2001 in Ghai et al., 2023). 'Without generalisation, there would be no evidence-based practice: research evidence can be used only if it has some relevance to settings and people outside of the contexts studied' (Polit & Beck, 2010; p. 1452). This results in the need to conduct research on orthorexia nervosa in a larger population to generalise findings across different groups.

Table 13.4  Directions for future research on orthorexia nervosa and the way forward

| Orthorexia nervosa | Future directions |
|---|---|
| *Conceptual issue* | |
| Definition | • The definition of orthorexia nervosa should be updated. For this reason, a conceptual review is needed. |
| Diagnostic criteria | • The inclusion of orthorexia nervosa in DSM would represent a significant advance in research and practice. |
| *Methodological issue* | |
| Diagnostic tool | • An assessment tool meant to diagnose orthorexia nervosa as well as to differentiate orthorexia nervosa from both normative healthy eating and anorexia nervosa is desirable and would be helpful. |
| *Research issue* | |
| Experimental and longitudinal studies | • These studies should be conducted with representative clinical and non-clinical samples. |
| Case studies | • To gain in-depth knowledge about patient(s) suffering from orthorexia nervosa. |
| Evidence-based research approach | • To ensure that studies of value on orthorexia nervosa are carried out by planning and designing new studies and placing new results in the context of the existing evidence (Robinson et al., 2021). |

In future studies, apart from the indicated future research directions (see Table 13.4), it would be worthwhile for researchers to address questions of generalisability in their samples explicitly, make data freely available (e.g. on Open Science Framework, Harvard Dataverse, Science Data Bank, Zenodo) to aid comparative research efforts, collect data broadly within their countries, as well as build partnerships with researchers (Wild, Kyröläinen & Kuperman, 2022).

Our views on orthorexia nervosa are amenable to continuous change based on new research data. The exploration of this phenomenon is needed not only because of its scientific value but, above all, because of its clinical value.

# References

Abdullah, M. A., Al Hourani, H. M., & Alkhatib, B. (2020). Prevalence of orthorexia nervosa among nutrition students and nutritionists: pilot study. *Clinical Nutrition ESPEN*, 40, 144–148.

Abraham, C., & Sheeran, P. (2005). The Health Belief Model. In M. Conner and P. Norman (Eds.), *Predicting Health Behaviour: Research and Practice with Social Cognition Models* (2nd Ed.). Maidenhead: Open University Press, pp. 28–80.

Adrogué, H. J., Tucker, B. M., & Madias, N. E. (2022). Diagnosis and management of hyponatremia: a review. *JAMA*, 328(3), 280–291.

Agopyan, A., Kenger, E. B., Kermen, S., Ulker, M. T., Uzsoy, M. A., & Yetgin, M. K. (2019). The relationship between orthorexia nervosa and body composition in female students of the nutrition and dietetics department. *Eating and Weight Disorders*, 24(2), 257–266.

Aiello, P., Toti, E., Villaño, D., Raguzzini, A., & Peluso, I. (2022). Overlap of orthorexia, eating attitude and psychological distress in some Italian and Spanish university students. *World Journal of Psychiatry*, 12(10), 1298–1312.

Aksoydan, E., & Camci, N. (2009). Prevalence of orthorexia nervosa among Turkish performance artists. *Eating and Weight Disorders*, 14(1), 33–37.

Albery, I. P., Shove, E., Bartlett, G., Frings, D., & Spada, M. M. (2022). Individual differences in selective attentional bias for healthy and unhealthy food-related stimuli and social identity as a vegan/vegetarian dissociate 'healthy' and 'unhealthy' orthorexia nervosa. *Appetite*, 178, 106261.

Alkerwi, A., Sauvageot, N., Malan, L., Shivappa, N., & Hébert, J. R. (2015). Association between nutritional awareness and diet quality: evidence from the observation of cardiovascular risk factors in Luxembourg (ORISCAV-LUX) study. *Nutrients*, 7(4), 2823–2838.

Allirot, X., Miragall, M., Perdices, I., Baños, R. M., Urdaneta, E., & Cebolla, A. (2018). Effects of a brief mindful eating induction on food choices and energy intake: external eating and mindfulness state as moderators. *Mindfulness*, 9(3), 750–760.

Almeida, C., Vieira Borba, V., & Santos, L. (2018). Orthorexia nervosa in a sample of Portuguese fitness participants. *Eating and Weight Disorders*, 23(4), 443–451.

Aloi, M., Moniaci, M., Rania, M., Carbone, E. A., Martino, G., Segura-Garcia, C., & Liuzza, M. T. (2023). Relationship between disgust and orthorexia nervosa and psychometric properties of the Italian Dusseldorf orthorexia scale in a general population sample. *Journal of Eating Disorders, 11*(1), 174.

Alvarenga, M. S., Martins, M. C., Sato, K. S., Vargas, S. V., Philippi, S. T., & Scagliusi, F. B. (2012). Orthorexia nervosa behavior in a sample of Brazilian dietitians assessed by the Portuguese version of ORTO-15. *Eating and Weight Disorders, 17*(1), e29–e35.

Alvarenga, M. D. S., Obara, A. A., Takeda, G. A., & Ferreira-Vivolo, S. R. G. (2022). Anti-fat attitudes of nutrition undergraduates in Brazil toward individuals with obesity. *Ciencia & Saude Coletiva, 27*(2), 747–760.

American Psychiatric Association. (2013). *Diagnostic and Statistical Manual of Mental Disorders* (5th Ed.). Arlington, VA: American Psychiatric Association.

American Psychiatric Association. (2021). *Guide to Submitting Proposals for Changes to DSM-5*. Arlington, VA: American Psychiatric Association.

American Psychiatric Association. (2022). *Diagnostic and Statistical Manual of Mental Disorders* (5th Ed., text rev.). Arlington, VA: American Psychiatric Association.

Anastasiades, E., & Argyrides, M. (2023). Exploring the role of positive body image in healthy orthorexia and orthorexia nervosa: a gender comparison. *Appetite, 185*, 106523.

Anderson, D. A., Donahue, J., Ehrlich, L. E., & Gorrell, S. (2018). Psychological assessment of the eating disorders. In W. S. Agras & A. Robinson (Eds.), *The Oxford Handbook of Eating Disorders*. Oxford: Oxford University Press, pp. 211–221.

Armstrong, D. (2009). Origins of the problem of health-related behaviours: a genealogical study. *Social Studies of Science, 39*(6), 909–926.

Arnett, J. J. (2008). The neglected 95%: why American psychology needs to become less American. *The American Psychologist, 63*(7), 602–614.

Asil, E., & Sürücüoğlu, M. S. (2015). Orthorexia nervosa in Turkish dietitians. *Ecology of Food and Nutrition, 54*(4), 303–313.

Atchison, A. E., & Zickgraf, H. F. (2022). Orthorexia nervosa and eating disorder behaviors: a systematic review of the literature. *Appetite, 177*, 106134.

Athanasaki, D., Lakoumentas, J., Feketea, G., & Vassilopoulou, E. (2023). The prevalence of orthorexia nervosa among Greek professional dancers. *Nutrients, 15*(2), 379.

Awad, E., Rogoza, R., Gerges, S., Obeid, S., & Hallit, S. (2022). Association of social media use disorder and orthorexia nervosa among Lebanese university students: the indirect effect of loneliness and factor structure of the

Social Media Use Disorder Short Form and the Jong-Gierveld Loneliness Scales. *Psychological Reports*, 332941221132985.

Azzi, R., Mhanna, M., Hallit, S., Obeid, S., & Soufia, M. (2023). Attachment styles and orthorexia nervosa among Lebanese adolescents: the indirect effect of self-esteem. *Archives de Pediatrie*, *30*(5), 314–320.

Babeau, C., Le Chevanton, T., Julien-Sweerts, S., Brochenin, A., Donini, L. M., & Fouques, D. (2020). Structural validation of the ORTO-12-FR questionnaire among a French sample as a first attempt to assess orthorexia nervosa in France. *Eating and Weight Disorders*, *25*(6), 1771–1778.

Bağci Bosi, A. T., Camur, D., & Güler, C. (2007). Prevalence of orthorexia nervosa in resident medical doctors in the faculty of medicine (Ankara, Turkey). *Appetite*, *49*(3), 661–666.

Bali, G., Kokka, I., Gonidakis, F., Papakonstantinou, E., Vlachakis, D., Chrousos, G. P., Kanaka-Gantenbein, C., & Bacopoulou, F. (2023). Validation of the Eating Habits Questionnaire in Greek adults. *EMBnet.journal*, *28*, e1029.

Balogh, E. P., Miller, B. T., Ball, J. R., Committee on Diagnostic Error in Health Care, Board on Health Care Services, Institute of Medicine, & The National Academies of Sciences, Engineering, and Medicine (Eds.). (2015). *Improving Diagnosis in Health Care*. Washington, DC: National Academies Press (US).

Banna, J. C., Gilliland, B., Keefe, M., & Zheng, D. (2016). Cross-cultural comparison of perspectives on healthy eating among Chinese and American undergraduate students. *BMC Public Health*, *16*(1), 1015.

Barnes, M. A., & Caltabiano, M. L. (2017). The interrelationship between orthorexia nervosa, perfectionism, body image and attachment style. *Eating and Weight Disorders*, *22*(1), 177–184.

Barnett, M. J., Dripps, W. R., & Blomquist, K. K. (2016). Organivore or organorexic? Examining the relationship between alternative food network engagement, disordered eating, and special diets. *Appetite*, *105*, 713–720.

Barrada, J. R., & Roncero, M. (2018). Bidimensional structure of the orthorexia: development and initial validation of a new instrument. *Anales de Psicología*, *34*(2), 283–291.

Bartel, S. J., Sherry, S. B., Farthing, G. R., & Stewart, S. H. (2020). Classification of orthorexia nervosa: further evidence for placement within the eating disorders spectrum. *Eating Behaviors*, *38*, 101406.

Barthels, F., Bamberg, L., & Pietrowsky, R. (2022). No elevated levels of orthorexic eating behavior in a sample of adults with allergies and food intolerances. *Eating and Weight Disorders*, *27*(8), 3781–3785.

Barthels, F., Barrada, J. R., & Roncero, M. (2019). Orthorexia nervosa and healthy orthorexia as new eating styles. *PloS One*, *14*(7), e0219609.

Barthels, F., Kisser, J., & Pietrowsky, R. (2021). Orthorexic eating behavior and body dissatisfaction in a sample of young females. *Eating and Weight Disorders, 26*(6), 2059–2063.

Barthels, F., Lavendel, S., Müller, R., & Pietrowsky, R. (2019). Relevance of orthorexic eating behavior in nutrition counseling and nutrition therapy. Results of a nationwide survey among German nutritionists. *Ernahrungs Umschau, 66*(12), 236–241.

Barthels F., Meyer F., & Pietrowsky R. (2015a). Orthorexic eating behavior. *Ernahrungs Umschau, 62*(10), 156–161.

Barthels, F., Meyer, F., & Pietrowsky, R. (2015b). Die Düsseldorfer Orthorexie Skala-Konstruktion und Evaluation eines Fragebogens zur Erfassung ortho-rektischen Ernährungsverhaltens [Düsseldorf Orthorexia Scale – construction and evaluation of a questionnaire measuring orthorexic eating behavior] *Zeitschrift für Klinische Psychologie und Psychotherapie, 44*(2), 97–105.

Barthels, F., Meyer, F., Huber, T., & Pietrowsky, R. (2017). Orthorexic eating behaviour as a coping strategy in patients with anorexia nervosa. *Eating and Weight Disorders, 22*(2), 269–276.

Barthels, F., Meyer, F., & Pietrowsky, R. (2018). Orthorexic and restrained eating behaviour in vegans, vegetarians, and individuals on a diet. *Eating and Weight Disorders, 23*, 159–166.

Barthels, F., Müller, R., Schüth, T., Friederich, H. C., & Pietrowsky, R. (2021). Orthorexic eating behavior in patients with somatoform disorders. *Eating and Weight Disorders, 26*(1), 135–143.

Bauer, S. M., Fusté, A., Andrés, A., & Saldaña, C. (2019). The Barcelona Orthorexia Scale (BOS): development process using the Delphi method. *Eating and Weight Disorders, 24*(2), 247–255.

Belloch, A., Roncero, M., & Perpiñá, C. (2016). Obsessional and eating disorder-related intrusive thoughts: differences and similarities within and between individuals vulnerable to OCD or to EDs. *European Eating Disorders Review, 24*(6), 446–454.

Bender D.A. (2009). *Dictionary of Food and Nutrition* (3rd Ed.). Oxford: Oxford University Press.

Bert, F., Gualano, M. R., Voglino, G., Rossello, P., Perret, J. P., & Siliquini, R. (2019). Orthorexia nervosa: a cross-sectional study among athletes competing in endurance sports in Northern Italy. *PloS One, 14*(8), e0221399.

Beshara, M., Hutchinson, A. D., & Wilson, C. (2013). Does mindfulness matter? Everyday mindfulness, mindful eating and self-reported serving size of energy dense foods among a sample of South Australian adults. *Appetite, 67*, 25–29.

Bhattacharya, A., Cooper, M., McAdams, C., Peebles, R., & Timko, C. A. (2022). Cultural shifts in the symptoms of anorexia nervosa: the case of orthorexia nervosa. *Appetite, 170*, 105869.

Billieux, J., Schimmenti, A., Khazaal, Y., Maurage, P., & Heeren, A. (2015). Are we overpathologizing everyday life? A tenable blueprint for behavioral addiction research. *Journal of Behavioral Addictions, 4*(3), 119–123.

Bisogni, C. A., Jastran, M., Seligson, M., & Thompson, A. (2012). How people interpret healthy eating: contributions of qualitative research. *Journal of Nutrition Education and Behavior, 44*(4), 282–301.

Bóna, E., Erdész, A., & Túry, F. (2021). Low self-esteem predicts orthorexia nervosa, mediated by spiritual attitudes among frequent exercisers. *Eating and Weight Disorders, 26*(8), 2481–2489.

Bóna, E., Túry, F., & Forgácsc, A. (2019). Evolutionary aspects of a new eating disorder: orthorexia nervosa in the 21st century. *Psychological Thought, 12*(2), 4–13.

Bonilla, D. A., Peralta-Alzate, J. O., Bonilla-Henao, J. A., Cannataro, R., Cardozo, L. A., Vargas-Molina, S., Stout, J. R., Kreider, R. B., & Petro, J. L. (2023). Insights into non-exercise physical activity on control of body mass: a review with practical recommendations. *Journal of Functional Morphology and Kinesiology, 8*(2), 44.

Bouchey, C., Ard, J., Bazzano, L., Heymsfield, S., Mayer-Davis, E., Sabaté, J., Snetselaar, L., Van Horn, L., Schneeman, B., English, L. K., Bates, M., Callahan, E., Venkatramanan, S., Butera, G., Terry, N., & Obbagy, J. (2020). Dietary patterns and all-cause mortality: a systematic review. US Department of Agriculture, Food and Nutrition Service, Center for Nutrition Policy and Promotion, Nutrition Evidence Systematic Review. https://doi.org/10.52570/NESR.DGAC2020.SR0108.

Bratman S. (1997). Health food junkie. *Yoga Journal*, September/October, 42–50.

Bratman S. (2017). Orthorexia vs. theories of healthy eating. *Eating and Weight Disorders, 22*(3), 381–385.

Bratman, S., & Knight, D. (2000). *Health Food Junkies: Orthorexia Nervosa: Overcoming the Obsession with Healthful Eating.* New York: Broadway.

Bridley, A., & Daffin, L. W. (2023). *Fundamentals of Psychological Disorders.* LibreTextsTM.

Brunett, K. M., & Oberle, C. D. (2022). The dark triad moderates the association between orthorexia nervosa and relationship (dis)satisfaction. *Eating and Weight Disorders, 27*(7), 2515–2521.

Brytek-Matera, A. (2012). Orthorexia nervosa – an eating disorder, obsessive-compulsive disorder or disturbed eating habit? *Archives of Psychiatry and Psychotherapy, 14*(1), 55–60.

Brytek-Matera, A. (2020a). Interaction between vegetarian versus omnivorous diet and unhealthy eating patterns (orthorexia nervosa, cognitive restraint) and body mass index in adults. *Nutrients, 12*(3), 646.

Brytek-Matera, A. (2020b). Restrained eating and vegan, vegetarian and omnivore dietary intakes. *Nutrients, 12*(7), 2133.

Brytek-Matera, A. (2021a). Vegetarian diet and orthorexia nervosa: a review of the literature. *Eating and Weight Disorders, 26*(1), 1–11.

Brytek-Matera, A. (2021b). The Polish version of the Düsseldorf Orthorexia Scale (PL-DOS) and its comparison with the English version of the DOS (E-DOS). *Eating and Weight Disorders, 26*(4), 1223–1232.

Brytek-Matera, A. (2023). Additional phenotypes of eating disorders: orthorexia nervosa. In: P. Robinson, T. Wade, B. Herpertz-Dahlmann, F. Fernandez-Aranda, J. Treasure, S. Wonderlich (Eds.), *Eating Disorders.* Cham: Springer.

Brytek-Matera, A., Czepczor-Bernat, K., Jurzak, H., Kornacka, M., & Kołodziejczyk, N. (2019). Strict health-oriented eating patterns (orthorexic eating behaviours) and their connection with a vegetarian and vegan diet. *Eating and Weight Disorders, 24*(3), 441–452.

Brytek-Matera, A., Donini, L. M., Krupa, M., Poggiogalle, E., & Hay, P. (2015a). Orthorexia nervosa and self-attitudinal aspects of body image in female and male university students. *Journal of Eating Disorders, 3*, 2.

Brytek-Matera, A., Donini, L. M., Krupa, M., Poggiogalle, E., & Hay, P. (2016). Erratum to: orthorexia nervosa and self-attitudinal aspects of body image in female and male university students. *Journal of Eating Disorders, 4*, 16.

Brytek-Matera, A., Fonte, M. L., Poggiogalle, E., Donini, L. M., & Cena, H. (2017). Orthorexia nervosa: relationship with obsessive-compulsive symptoms, disordered eating patterns and body uneasiness among Italian university students. *Eating and Weight Disorders, 22*(4), 609–617.

Brytek-Matera, A., Krupa, M., Poggiogalle, E., & Donini, L. M. (2014). Adaptation of the ORTHO-15 test to Polish women and men. *Eating and Weight Disorders, 19*(1), 69–76.

Brytek-Matera, A., Obeid, S., Donini, L. M., Rogoza, M., Marchlewska, M., Plichta, M., Jezewska-Zychowicz, M., Hallit, S., & Rogoza, R. (2023). Psychometric properties of the ORTO-R in a community-based sample of women and men from Poland. *Journal of Eating Disorders, 11*(1), 9.

Brytek-Matera, A., Onieva-Zafra, M. D., Parra-Fernández, M. L., Staniszewska, A., Modrzejewska, J., & Fernández-Martínez, E. (2020a). Evaluation of orthorexia nervosa and symptomatology associated with eating disorders among European university students: a multicentre cross-sectional study. *Nutrients, 12*(12), 3716.

Brytek-Matera, A., Pardini, S., Modrzejewska, J., Modrzejewska, A., Szymańska, P., Czepczor-Bernat, K., & Novara, C. (2022). Orthorexia nervosa and its association with obsessive-compulsive disorder symptoms: initial cross-cultural comparison between Polish and Italian university students. *Eating and Weight Disorders*, *27*(3), 913–927.

Brytek-Matera, A., Plasonja, N., & Décamps, G. (2020). Assessing orthorexia nervosa: validation of the Polish version of the Eating Habits Questionnaire in a general population sample. *Nutrients*, *12*(12), 3820.

Brytek-Matera, A., Rogoza, R., Gramaglia, C., & Zeppegno, P. (2015b). Predictors of orthorexic behaviours in patients with eating disorders: a preliminary study. *BMC Psychiatry*, *15*, 252.

Brytek-Matera, A., Sacre, H., Staniszewska, A., & Hallit, S. (2020b). The prevalence of orthorexia nervosa in Polish and Lebanese adults and its relationship with sociodemographic variables and BMI ranges: a cross-cultural perspective. *Nutrients*, *12*(12), 3865.

Brytek-Matera, A., Staniszewska, A., & Hallit, S. (2020c). Identifying the profile of orthorexic behavior and 'normal' eating behavior with cluster analysis: a cross-sectional study among Polish adults. *Nutrients*, *12*(11), 3490.

Bucchianeri, M. M., Arikian, A. J., Hannan, P. J., Eisenberg, M. E., & Neumark-Sztainer, D. (2013). Body dissatisfaction from adolescence to young adulthood: findings from a 10-year longitudinal study. *Body Image*, *10*(1), 1–7.

Bundros, J., Clifford, D., Silliman, K., & Neyman Morris, M. (2016). Prevalence of orthorexia nervosa among college students based on Bratman's test and associated tendencies. *Appetite*, *101*, 86–94.

Burger, M. K., & Schaller, D.J. Metabolic acidosis. [Updated 17 July 2023]. In: StatPearls [Internet]. Treasure Island (FL): StatPearls Publishing; 2023 January. www.ncbi.nlm.nih.gov/books/NBK482146/.

Burlingame, B., & Dernini, S. (2012). *Sustainable Diets and Biodiversity Directions and Solutions for Policy, Research And Action*. Rome: FAO Headquarters.

Busatta, D., Cassioli, E., Rossi, E., Campanino, C., Ricca, V., & Rotella, F. (2022). Orthorexia among patients with eating disorders, student dietitians and general population: a pilot study. *Eating and Weight Disorders*, *27*(2), 847–851.

Caferoglu, Z., & Toklu, H. (2022). Orthorexia nervosa in Turkish dietitians and dietetic students. *L'Encephale*, *48*(1), 13–19.

Calugi, S., Dalle Grave, R., Sartirana, M., & Fairburn, C. G. (2015). Time to restore body weight in adults and adolescents receiving cognitive behaviour therapy for anorexia nervosa. *Journal of Eating Disorders*, *3*, 21.

Cambridge Dictionary. https://dictionary.cambridge.org/dictionary/english/mania.

Cartwright, M. M. (2004). Eating disorder emergencies: understanding the medical complexities of the hospitalized eating disordered patient. *Critical Care Nursing Clinics of North America*, *16*(4), 515–530.

Cena, H., Barthels, F., Cuzzolaro, M., Bratman, S., Brytek-Matera, A., Dunn, T., Varga, M., Missbach, B., & Donini, L. M. (2019). Definition and diagnostic criteria for orthorexia nervosa: a narrative review of the literature. *Eating and Weight Disorders*, *24*(2), 209–246.

Cerea, S., Bottesi, G., Pacelli, Q. F., Paoli, A., & Ghisi, M. (2018). Muscle dysmorphia and its associated psychological features in three groups of recreational athletes. *Scientific Reports*, *8*(1), 8877.

Cerolini, S., Vacca, M., Zagaria, A., Donini, L. M., Barbaranelli, C., & Lombardo, C. (2022). Italian adaptation of the Düsseldorf Orthorexia Scale (I-DOS): psychometric properties and prevalence of orthorexia nervosa among an Italian sample. *Eating and Weight Disorders*, *27*(4), 1405–1413.

Chace, S., & Kluck, A. S. (2022). Validation of the Teruel Orthorexia Scale and relationship to health anxiety in a US sample. *Eating and Weight Disorders*, *27*(4), 1437–1447.

Chaki, B., Pal, S., & Bandyopadhyay, A. (2013). Exploring scientific legitimacy of orthorexia nervosa: a newly emerging eating disorder. *Journal of Human Sport and Exercise*, *8*(4), 1045–1053.

Chard, C. A., Hilzendegen, C., Barthels, F., & Stroebele-Benschop, N. (2019). Psychometric evaluation of the English version of the Düsseldorf Orthorexie Scale (DOS) and the prevalence of orthorexia nervosa among a US student sample. *Eating and Weight Disorders*, *24*(2), 275–281.

Chen, P. J., & Antonelli, M. (2020). Conceptual models of food choice: influential factors related to foods, individual differences, and society. *Foods*, *9*(12), 1898.

Cheshire, A., Berry, M., & Fixsen, A. (2020). What are the key features of orthorexia nervosa and influences on its development? A qualitative investigation. *Appetite*, *155*, 104798.

Chiavaroli, L., Viguiliouk, E., Nishi, S. K., Blanco Mejia, S., Rahelić, D., Kahleová, H., Salas-Salvadó, J., Kendall, C. W., & Sievenpiper, J. L. (2019). DASH dietary pattern and cardiometabolic outcomes: an umbrella review of systematic reviews and meta-analyses. *Nutrients*, *11*(2), 338.

Cho, H.-B., & Hyun, M.-H. (2020). Orthorexia nervosa, fear of obesity. *Stress*, *28*, 68–75.

Çiçekoğlu, P., & Tunçay, G. Y. (2018). A comparison of eating attitudes between vegans/vegetarians and nonvegans/nonvegetarians in terms of orthorexia nervosa. *Archives of Psychiatric Nursing*, *32*(2), 200–205.

Clifford, T., & Blyth, C. (2019). A pilot study comparing the prevalence of orthorexia nervosa in regular students and those in university sports teams. *Eating and Weight Disorders*, *24*(3), 473–480.

Colao, A., Vetrani, C., Muscogiuri, G., Barrea, L., Tricopoulou, A., Soldati, L., Piscitelli, P., & UNESCO Chair on Health Education and Sustainable Development (2022). 'Planeterranean' Diet: extending worldwide the health benefits of Mediterranean Diet based on nutritional properties of locally available foods. *Journal of Translational Medicine*, *20*(1), 232.

Conner, M., & Norman, P. (2005). *Predicting and Changing Health Behaviour: Research and Practice with Social Cognition Models*. McGraw-Hill Education.

Conner, M. (2019). Models of Health Behaviour. In Llewellyn, C., Susan, A., McManus, C., Newman, S., Petrie, K. J., Revenson, T. A., & Weinman, J. (eds.), *Cambridge Handbook of Psychology, Health and Medicine* (pp. 55–60). Cambridge University Press.

Cori, G.D.C, Petty, M. L. B., & Alvarenga, M. dos S. (2015) Atitudes de nutricionistas em relação a indivíduos obesos – um estudo exploratório [Attitudes of dietitians in relation to obese individuals – an exploratory study]. *Ciência & Saúde Coletiva*, *20*(2), 565–576.

Cosentino, C., Rossi, E., Pala, L., Lelmi, R., Campanino, C., Ricca, V., Mannucci, E., Dicembrini, I., & Rotella, F. (2023). Orthorexia nervosa and type 1 diabetes: results of a cross-sectional study. *Acta Diabetologica*, *60*(5), 681–686.

Cosh, S. M., Olson, J., & Tully, P. J. (2023). Exploration of orthorexia nervosa and diagnostic overlap with eating disorders, anorexia nervosa and obsessive-compulsive disorder. *International Journal of Eating Disorders*, 10.1002/ eat.24051. Advance online publication.

Costa, C. B., & Hardan-Khalil, K. (2019). Orthorexia nervosa and obsessive-compulsive behavior among college students in the United States. *Journal of Nursing Education and Practice*, *9*(2), 67.

Costanzo, G., Marchetti, D., Manna, G., Verrocchio, M. C., & Falgares, G. (2022). The role of eating disorders features, psychopathology, and defense mechanisms in the comprehension of orthorexic tendencies. *Eating and Weight Disorders*, *27*(7), 2713–2724.

Crawford, R. (1980). Healthism and the medicalization of everyday life. *International Journal of Health Services*, *10*(3), 365–388.

Cuzzolaro, M., & Donini, L. M. (2016). Orthorexia nervosa by proxy? *Eating and Weight Disorders*, *21*(4), 549–551.

Dalgleish, T., Black, M., Johnston, D., & Bevan, A. (2020). Transdiagnostic approaches to mental health problems: current status and future directions. *Journal of Consulting and Clinical Psychology*, *88*(3), 179–195.

Dalle Grave, R., Calugi, S., Doll, H. A., & Fairburn, C. G. (2013). Enhanced cognitive behaviour therapy for adolescents with anorexia nervosa: an alternative to family therapy? *Behaviour Research and Therapy, 51*(1), R9-r12.

Davis, R., Campbell, R., Hildon, Z., Hobbs, L., & Michie, S. (2015). Theories of behaviour and behaviour change across the social and behavioural sciences: a scoping review. *Health Psychology Review, 9*(3), 323–344.

Dell'Osso, L., Abelli, M., Carpita, B., Pini, S., Castellini, G., Carmassi, C., & Ricca, V. (2016). Historical evolution of the concept of anorexia nervosa and relationships with orthorexia nervosa, autism, and obsessive-compulsive spectrum. *Neuropsychiatric Disease and Treatment, 12*, 1651–1660.

Demirer, B., Yardımcı, H. (2024). Is mindful eating higher in individuals with orthorexia nervosa? A cross-sectional study. *Journal of Public Health.* https://doi.org/10.1007/s10389-023-01829-0.

Depa, J., Barrada, J. R., & Roncero, M. (2019). Are the motives for food choices different in orthorexia nervosa and healthy orthorexia? *Nutrients, 11*(3), 697.

Depa, J., Schweizer, J., Bekers, S. K., Hilzendegen, C., & Stroebele-Benschop, N. (2017). Prevalence and predictors of orthorexia nervosa among German students using the 21-item-DOS. *Eating and Weight Disorders, 22*(1), 193–199.

Derbyshire, E. J. (2017). Flexitarian diets and health: a review of the evidence-based literature. *Frontiers in Nutrition, 3*, 55.

Dietary Guidelines Advisory Committee (2015). Scientific Report of the 2015 Dietary Guidelines Advisory Committee: Advisory Report to the Secretary of Health and Human Services and the Secretary of Agriculture. Washington, DC : US Department of Agriculture, Agricultural Research Service.

Domingues, R. B., & Carmo, C. (2021). Orthorexia nervosa in yoga practitioners: relationship with personality, attitudes about appearance, and yoga engagement. *Eating and Weight Disorders, 26*(3), 789–795.

Donini, L. M., Marsili, D., Graziani, M. P., Imbriale, M., & Cannella, C. (2004). Orthorexia nervosa: a preliminary study with a proposal for diagnosis and an attempt to measure the dimension of the phenomenon. *Eating and Weight Disorders, 9*(2), 151–157.

Donini, L. M., Marsili, D., Graziani, M. P., Imbriale, M., & Cannella, C. (2005). Orthorexia nervosa: validation of a diagnosis questionnaire. *Eating and Weight Disorders, 10*(2), e28–e32.

Donini, L. M., Barrada, J. R., Barthels, F., Dunn, T. M., Babeau, C., Brytek-Matera, A., Cena, H., Cerolini, S., Cho, H. H., Coimbra, M., Cuzzolaro, M., Ferreira, C., Galfano, V., Grammatikopoulou, M. G., Hallit, S., Håman, L., Hay, P., Jimbo, M., Lasson, C., Lindgren, E. C., … Lombardo, C. (2022).

A consensus document on definition and diagnostic criteria for orthorexia nervosa. *Eating and Weight Disorders*, *27*(8), 3695–3711.

Douma, E. R., Valente, M., & Syurina, E. V. (2021). Developmental pathway of orthorexia nervosa: factors contributing to progression from healthy eating to excessive preoccupation with healthy eating. Experiences of Dutch health professionals. *Appetite*, *158*, 105008.

Drescher, J. (2015). Queer diagnoses revisited: the past and future of homosexuality and gender diagnoses in DSM and ICD. *International Review of Psychiatry*, *27*(5), 386–395.

D'Urso, G., Maynard, A., Lionetti, F., Spinelli, M., & Fasolo, M. (2023). Parental relationships, emotion regulation and orthorexia: a study on adolescent athletes. *Nutrition and Health*, 2601060231194825. Advance online publication.

DuBois, H., Rodgers, R. F., Franko, D. L., Eddy, K. T., & Thomas, J. J. (2017). A network analysis investigation of the cognitive-behavioral theory of eating disorders. *Behaviour Research and Therapy*, *97*, 213–221.

Duradoni, M., Gursesli, M. C., Fiorenza, M., & Guazzini, A. (2023). The relationship between orthorexia nervosa and obsessive compulsive disorder. *European Journal of Investigation in Health, Psychology and Education*, *13*(5), 861–869.

Dunn, T. M., & Bratman, S. (2016). On orthorexia nervosa: a review of the literature and proposed diagnostic criteria. *Eating Behaviors*, *21*, 11–17.

Dunn, T. M., Gibbs, J., Whitney, N., & Starosta, A. (2017). Prevalence of orthorexia nervosa is less than 1%: data from a US sample. *Eating and Weight Disorders*, *22*(1), 185–192.

Eertmans, A., Baeyens, F., & Van den Bergh, O. (2001). Food likes and their relative importance in human eating behavior: review and preliminary suggestions for health promotion. *Health Education Research*, *16*(4), 443–456.

Elias, M. C., Gomes, D. L., & Paracampo, C. C. P. (2022). Associations between orthorexia nervosa, body self-image, nutritional beliefs, and behavioral rigidity. *Nutrients*, *14*(21), 4578.

Elran-Barak, R., Sztainer, M., Goldschmidt, A. B., Crow, S. J., Peterson, C. B., Hill, L. L., … & Le Grange, D. (2015). Dietary restriction behaviors and binge eating in anorexia nervosa, bulimia nervosa and binge eating disorder: trans-diagnostic examination of the restraint model. *Eating Behaviors*, *18*, 192–196.

Eriksson, L., Baigi, A., Marklund, B., & Lindgren, E. C. (2008). Social physique anxiety and sociocultural attitudes toward appearance impact on orthorexia test in fitness participants. *Scandinavian Journal of Medicine & Science in Sports*, *18*(3), 389–394.

Eskandari, A., Naeimi, M., Fathi-Ashtiani, A., & Farahani, H. (2022). Psychometric properties of the Persian version of the Orthorexia Nervosa Scale (ORTO-15). *Quarterly Journal of Health Psychology, 11*(43), 21–40.

European Commission (2023). *Reformulating our food for a healthier life*. https://knowledge4policy.ec.europa.eu/blog/reformulating-our-food-healthier-life%E2%80%%AF_en.

European Food Safety Authority (EFSA; 2010). *Scientific Opinion on Establishing Food-Based Dietary Guidelines*, EFSA Panel on Dietetic Products, Nutrition, and Allergies (NDA).

Fairburn, C. G. (2008). *Cognitive Behavior Therapy and Eating Disorders*. New York: Guilford Press.

Fairburn, C. G., Bailey-Straebler, S., Basden, S., Doll, H. A., Jones, R., Murphy, R., ... Cooper, Z. (2015). A transdiagnostic comparison of enhanced cognitive behaviour therapy (CBT-E) and interpersonal psychotherapy in the treatment of eating disorders. *Behaviour Research and Therapy, 70*, 64–71.

Fairburn, C. G., Cooper, Z., Doll, H. A., O'Connor, M. E., Palmer, R. L., & Dalle Grave, R. (2013). Enhanced cognitive behaviour therapy for adults with anorexia nervosa: a UK-Italy study. *Behaviour Research and Therapy, 51*(1), R2-8.

Fairburn, C. G., Cooper, Z., Doll, H. A., & Welch, S. L. (1999). Risk factors for anorexia nervosa: three integrated case-control comparisons. *Archives of General Psychiatry, 56*(5), 468–476.

Fairburn, C. G., Cooper, Z., & Shafran, R. (2003). Cognitive behaviour therapy for eating disorders: A 'transdiagnostic' theory and treatment. *Behaviour Research and Therapy, 41*, 509–528.

Falgares, G., Costanzo, G., Manna, G., Marchetti, D., Barrada, J. R., Roncero, M., Verrocchio, M. C., & Ingoglia, S. (2023). Healthy orthorexia vs. orthorexia nervosa: Italian validation of the Teruel Orthorexia Scale (TOS). *Eating and Weight Disorders, 28*(1), 42.

Fallon, E. A., Harris, B. S., & Johnson, P. (2014). Prevalence of body dissatisfaction among a United States adult sample. *Eating Behaviors, 15*(1), 151–158.

FAO (Food and Agriculture Organization of the United Nations; 2012). *Sustainable Diets and Biodiversity: Directions and Solutions for Policy, Research and Action*. Rome.

FAO (2015). Food-based dietary guidelines. www.fao.org/nutrition/nutrition-education/food-dietary-guidelines/en/.

FAO and WHO (2019). *Sustainable Healthy Diets – Guiding Principles*. Rome.

Farrar, S. T., Plagnol, A. C., & Tapper, K. (2022). The effect of priming on food choice: a field and laboratory study. *Appetite, 168*, 105749.

Ferreira, C., & Coimbra, M. (2021). To further understand orthorexia nervosa: DOS validity for the Portuguese population and its relationship with psychological indicators, sex, BMI and dietary pattern. *Eating and Weight Disorders*, *26*(7), 2127–2134.

Fineberg, N. A., Menchon, J. M., Zohar, J., & Veltman, D. J. (2016). Compulsivity: a new trans-diagnostic research domain for the Roadmap for Mental Health Research in Europe (ROAMER) and Research Domain Criteria (RDoC) initiatives. *European Neuropsychopharmacology*, *26*(5), 797–799.

Fixsen, A., Cheshire, A., & Berry, M. (2020). The social construction of a concept-orthorexia nervosa: morality narratives and psycho-politics. *Qualitative Health Research*, *30*(7), 1101–1113.

Foot, H., & Sanford, A. (2004). The use and abuse of student participants. *The Psychologist*, *17*(5), 256–259.

Foyster, M., Sultan, N., Tonkovic, M. Govus, Burton-Murray, H., Tuck, C. J., & Biesiekierski, J. R. (2023). Assessing the presence and motivations of orthorexia nervosa among athletes and adults with eating disorders: a cross-sectional study. *Eating and Weight Disorders*, 28, 101. https://doi.org/10.1007/s40519-023-01631-7.

Freedman, L. S., Commins, J. M., Moler, J. E., Arab, L., Baer, D. J., Kipnis, V., Midthune, D., Moshfegh, A. J., Neuhouser, M. L., Prentice, R. L., Schatzkin, A., Spiegelman, D., Subar, A. F., Tinker, L. F., & Willett, W. (2014). Pooled results from 5 validation studies of dietary self-report instruments using recovery biomarkers for energy and protein intake. *American Journal of Epidemiology*, *180*(2), 172–188.

Freeland-Graves, J. H., Nitzke, S., & Academy of Nutrition and Dietetics (2013). Position of the academy of nutrition and dietetics: total diet approach to healthy eating. *Journal of the Academy of Nutrition and Dietetics*, *113*(2), 307–317.

Freire, G. L. M., da Silva Paulo, J. R., da Silva, A. A., Batista, R. P. R., Alves, J. F. N., & do Nascimento Junior, J. R. A. (2020). Body dissatisfaction, addiction to exercise and risk behaviour for eating disorders among exercise practitioners. *Journal of Eating Disorders*, 8, 23.

Forouzanfar, M.H., Alexander, L., Anderson, H.R., Bachman, V.F., Biryukov, S., Brauer, M., Burnett, R., Casey, D., Coates, M.M., Cohen, A. & Delwiche, K. 2015. Global, regional, and national comparative risk assessment of 79 behavioural, environmental and occupational, and metabolic risks or clusters of risks in 188 countries, 1990–2013: a systematic analysis for the Global Burden of Disease Study 2013. *Lancet*, *386*(10010), 2287–2323.

Fusar-Poli, P., Solmi, M., Brondino, N., Davies, C., Chae, C., Politi, P., Borgwardt, S., Lawrie, S. M., Parnas, J., & McGuire, P. (2019). Transdiagnostic psychiatry: a systematic review. *World Psychiatry: Official Journal of the World Psychiatric Association (WPA), 18*(2), 192–207.

GBD 2013 Risk Factors Collaborators, Forouzanfar, M. H., Alexander, L., Anderson, H. R., Bachman, V. F., Biryukov, S., Brauer, M., Burnett, R., Casey, D., Coates, M. M., Cohen, A., Delwiche, K., Estep, K., Frostad, J. J., Astha, K. C., Kyu, H. H., Moradi-Lakeh, M., Ng, M., Slepak, E. L., Thomas, B. A., ... & Murray, C. J. (2015). Global, regional, and national comparative risk assessment of 79 behavioural, environmental and occupational, and metabolic risks or clusters of risks in 188 countries, 1990–2013: a systematic analysis for the Global Burden of Disease Study 2013. *Lancet, 386*(10010), 2287–2323.

Gearhardt, A. N., Corbin, W. R., & Brownell, K. D. (2009). Food addiction: an examination of the diagnostic criteria for dependence. *Journal of Addiction Medicine, 3*(1), 1–7.

Gerontidis, A., Grammatikopoulou, M. G., Tzimos, C., Gkiouras, K., Taousani, E., Athanasiadis, L., & Goulis, D. G. (2022). Effectors of pregorexia and emesis among pregnant women: a pilot study. *Nutrients, 14*(24), 5275.

Ghai, S., Fassi, L., Awadh, F., & Orben, A. (2023). Lack of sample diversity in research on adolescent depression and social media use: a scoping review and meta-analysis. *Clinical Psychological Science, 11*(5), 759–772.

Gkiouras, K., Grammatikopoulou, M. G., Tsaliki, T., Ntwali, L., Nigdelis, M. P., Gerontidis, A., Taousani, E., Tzimos, C., Rogoza, R., Bogdanos, D. P., Donini, L. M., & Goulis, D. G. (2022). Orthorexia nervosa: replication and validation of the ORTO questionnaires translated into Greek in a survey of 848 Greek individuals. *Hormones (Athens, Greece), 21*(2), 251–260.

Gleaves, D. H., Graham, E. C., & Ambwani, S. (2013). Measuring 'orthorexia': development of the Eating Habits Questionnaire. *The International Journal of Educational and Psychological Assessment, 12*(2), 1–18.

Global Nutrition Report (2020). https://globalnutritionreport.org/reporst/2020-global-nutrition-report.

Gnanaraj, J., Parnes, A., Francis, C. W., Go, R. S., Takemoto, C. M., & Hashmi, S. K. (2018). Approach to pancytopenia: diagnostic algorithm for clinical hematologists. *Blood Reviews, 32*(5), 361–367.

Gochman, D. S. (Ed.). (1997). *Handbook of Health Behavior Research*. New York: Plenum.

Godefroy, V., Trinchera, L., & Dorard, G. (2021). Optimizing the empirical assessment of orthorexia nervosa through EHQ and clarifying its relationship with BMI. *Eating and Weight Disorders, 26*(2), 649–659.

Gonidakis, F., Poulopoulou, C., Michopoulos, I., & Varsou, E. (2021). Validation of the Greek ORTO-15 questionnaire for the assessment of orthorexia nervosa and its relation to eating disorders symptomatology. *Eating and Weight Disorders, 26*(8), 2471–2479.

Gorrasi, I. S. R., Bonetta, S., Roppolo, M., Abbate Daga, G., Bo, S., Tagliabue, A., Ferraris, C., Guglielmetti, M., Arpesella, M., Gaeta, M., Gallé, F., Di Onofrio, V., Liguori, F., Liguori, G., Gilli, G., & Carraro, E. (2020). Traits of orthorexia nervosa and muscle dysmorphia in Italian university students: a multicentre study. *Eating and Weight Disorders, 25*(5), 1413–1423.

Gorrasi, I. S. R., Ferraris, C., Degan, R., Daga, G. A., Bo, S., Tagliabue, A., Guglielmetti, M., Roppolo, M., Gilli, G., Maran, D. A., & Carraro, E. (2022). Use of online and paper-and-pencil questionnaires to assess the distribution of orthorexia nervosa, muscle dysmorphia and eating disorders among university students: can different approaches lead to different results? *Eating and Weight Disorders, 27*(3), 989–999.

Gramaglia, C., Brytek-Matera, A., Rogoza, R., & Zeppegno, P. (2017). Orthorexia and anorexia nervosa: two distinct phenomena? A cross-cultural comparison of orthorexic behaviours in clinical and non-clinical samples. *BMC Psychiatry, 17*(1), 75.

Gramaglia, C., Gambaro, E., Delicato, C., Marchetti, M., Sarchiapone, M., Ferrante, D., Roncero, M., Perpiñá, C., Brytek-Matera, A., Wojtyna, E., & Zeppegno, P. (2019). Orthorexia nervosa, eating patterns and personality traits: a cross-cultural comparison of Italian, Polish and Spanish university students. *BMC Psychiatry, 19*(1), 235.

Gramaglia, C., Gattoni, E., Ferrante, D., Abbate-Daga, G., Baldissera, E., Calugi, S., Cascino, G., Castellini, G., Collantoni, E., Favaro, A., Marzola, E., Monteleone, A. M., Monteleone, P., Oriani, M. G., Renna, C., Ricca, V., Salvo, P., Santonastaso, P., Segura-Garcia, C., Volpe, U., … Zeppegno, P. (2022). What do Italian healthcare professionals think about orthorexia nervosa? Results from a multicenter survey. *Eating and Weight Disorders, 27*(6), 2037–2049.

Grammatikopoulou, M. G., Gkiouras, K., Markaki, A., Theodoridis, X., Tsakiri, V., Mavridis, P., Dardavessis, T., & Chourdakis, M. (2018). Food addiction, orthorexia, and food-related stress among dietetics students. *Eating and Weight Disorders, 23*(4), 459–467.

Gratz, K. L., & Roemer, L. (2004). Multidimensional assessment of emotion regulation and dysregulation: development, factor structure, and initial validation of the difficulties in emotion regulation scale. *Journal of Psychopathology and Behavioral Assessment, 26*(1), 41–54.

Green H. (2015). Should foods or nutrients be the focus of guidelines to promote healthful eating? *Nutrition Bulletin, 40*(4), 296–302.

Greetfeld, M., Hessler-Kaufmann, J. B., Brandl, B., Skurk, T., Holzapfel, C., Quadflieg, N., Schlegl, S., Hauner, H., & Voderholzer, U. (2021). Orthorexic tendencies in the general population: association with demographic data, psychiatric symptoms, and utilization of mental health services. *Eating and Weight Disorders*, *26*(5), 1511–1519.

Greville-Harris, M., Smithson, J., & Karl, A. (2020). What are people's experiences of orthorexia nervosa? A qualitative study of online blogs. *Eating and Weight Disorders*, *25*(6), 1693–1702.

Greville-Harris, M., Talbot, C. V., Moseley, R. L., & Vuillier, L. (2022). Conceptualisations of health in orthorexia nervosa: a mixed-methods study. *Eating and Weight Disorders*, *27*(8), 3135–3143.

Grilo, C. M., & Masheb, R. M. (2000). Onset of dieting vs. binge eating in outpatients with binge eating disorder. *International Journal of Obesity*, *24*(4), 404–409.

Gross, J. J. (1998). The emerging field of emotion regulation: an integrative review. *Review of General Psychology*, *2*(3), 271–299.

Guglielmetti, M., Ferraro, O. E., Gorrasi, I. S. R., Carraro, E., Bo, S., Abbate-Daga, G., Tagliabue, A., & Ferraris, C. (2022). Lifestyle-related risk factors of orthorexia can differ among the students of distinct university courses. *Nutrients*, *14*(5), 1111.

Hachem, F., Capone, R., Yannakoulia, M., Dernini, S., Hwalla, N. & Kalaitzidis, C. (2016). The Mediterranean diet: a sustainable consumption pattern. In FAO and CIHEAM. Mediterra 2016. Zero Waste in the Mediterranean. Natural Resources, Food and Knowledge, pp. 243–261. Paris, Presses de Sciences Po.

Haddad, C., Hallit, R., Akel, M., Honein, K., Akiki, M., Kheir, N., Obeid, S., & Hallit, S. (2020). Validation of the Arabic version of the ORTO-15 questionnaire in a sample of the Lebanese population. *Eating and Weight Disorders*, *25*(4), 951–960

Haddad, C., Obeid, S., Akel, M., Honein, K., Akiki, M., Azar, J., & Hallit, S. (2019). Correlates of orthorexia nervosa among a representative sample of the Lebanese population. *Eating and Weight Disorders*, *24*(3), 481–493.

Hafstad, S. M., Bauer, J., Harris, A., & Pallesen, S. (2023). The prevalence of orthorexia in exercising populations: a systematic review and meta-analysis. *Journal of Eating Disorders*, *11*(1), 15.

Hallit, S., Azzi, V., Malaeb, D., & Obeid, S. (2022). Any overlap between orthorexia nervosa and obsessive-compulsive disorder in Lebanese adults? Results of a cross-sectional study and validation of the 12-item and 4-item obsessive-compulsive inventory (OCI-12 and OCI-4). *BMC Psychiatry*, *22*(1), 470.

Hallit, S., Barrada, J. R., Salameh, P., Sacre, H., Roncero, M., & Obeid, S. (2021). The relation of orthorexia with lifestyle habits: Arabic versions of the Eating Habits Questionnaire and the Dusseldorf Orthorexia Scale. *Journal of Eating Disorders, 9*(1), 102.

Hallit, S., Brytek-Matera, A., & Obeid, S. (2021). Orthorexia nervosa and disordered eating attitudes among Lebanese adults: assessing psychometric proprieties of the ORTO-R in a population-based sample. *PloS One, 16*(8), e0254948.

Håman, L., Lindgren, E. C., & Prell, H. (2017). 'If it's not Iron it's Iron f*cking biggest Ironman': personal trainers's views on health norms, orthorexia and deviant behaviours. *International Journal of Qualitative Studies on Health and Well-being, 12*(1), 1364602.

Hanel, P. H., & Vione, K. C. (2016). Do student samples provide an accurate estimate of the general public? *PloS One, 11*(12), e0168354.

Harrison, M. R., Palma, G., Buendia, T., Bueno-Tarodo, M., Quell, D., & Hachem, F. (2022). A scoping review of indicators for sustainable healthy diets. *Frontiers in Sustainable Food Systems, 5*, 822263.

Hastings, S. (2012). *The Secret lives of Somerset Maugham: A Biography*. Simon and Schuster.

Havigerová, J. M., Dosedlová, J., & Burešová, I. (2018). One health behavior or many health-related behaviors? *Psychology Research and Behavior Management, 12*, 23–30.

Hay P. (2020). Current approach to eating disorders: a clinical update. *Internal Medicine Journal, 50*(1), 24–29.

Hay P. (2021). Is orthorexia nervosa a healthy way of being or a mental health disorder? Commentary on He et al. (2020). *International Journal of Eating Disorders, 54*(2), 222–224.

Hay, P., Chinn, D., Forbes, D., Madden, S., Newton, R., Sugenor, L., Touyz, S., Ward, W., & Royal Australian and New Zealand College of Psychiatrists (2014). Royal Australian and New Zealand College of Psychiatrists clinical practice guidelines for the treatment of eating disorders. *The Australian and New Zealand Journal of Psychiatry, 48*(11), 977–1008.

Hayes, O., Wu, M. S., De Nadai, A. S., & Storch, E. A. (2017). Orthorexia nervosa: an examination of the prevalence, correlates, and associated impairment in a university sample. *Journal of Cognitive Psychotherapy, 31*(2), 124–135.

Hanganu-Bresch C. (2020). Orthorexia: eating right in the context of healthism. *Medical Humanities, 46*(3), 311–322.

Håman, L., Barker-Ruchti, N., Patriksson, G., & Lindgren, E. C. (2015). Orthorexia nervosa: an integrative literature review of a lifestyle syndrome.

*International Journal of Qualitative Studies on Health and Well-Being, 10,* 26799.

Håman, L., Lindgren, E. C., & Prell, H. (2017). 'If it's not Iron it's Iron f*cking biggest Ironman': personal trainers's views on health norms, orthorexia and deviant behaviours. *International Journal of Qualitative Studies on Health and Well-being, 12*(1), 1364602.

He, J., Ma, H., Barthels, F., & Fan, X. (2019). Psychometric properties of the Chinese version of the Düsseldorf Orthorexia Scale: prevalence and demographic correlates of orthorexia nervosa among Chinese university students. *Eating and Weight Disorders, 24*(3), 453–463.

He, J., Zhao, Y., Zhang, H., & Lin, Z. (2021). Orthorexia nervosa is associated with positive body image and life satisfaction in Chinese elderly: evidence for a positive psychology perspective. *International Journal of Eating Disorders, 54*(2), 212–221.

Heiss, S., Coffino, J. A., & Hormes, J. M. (2019). What does the ORTO-15 measure? Assessing the construct validity of a common orthorexia nervosa questionnaire in a meat avoiding sample. *Appetite, 135,* 93–99.

Hemler, E. C., & Hu, F. B. (2019). Plant-based diets for personal, population, and planetary health. *Advances in Nutrition, 10*(Suppl_4), S275–S283.

Hepworth K. (2010). Eating disorders today – not just a girl thing. *Journal of Christian Nursing: a quarterly publication of Nurses Christian Fellowship, 27*(3), 236–243.

Hessler-Kaufmann, J. B., Meule, A., Greetfeld, M., Schlegl, S., & Voderholzer, U. (2021). Orthorexic tendencies in inpatients with mental disorders. *Journal of Psychosomatic Research, 140,* 110317.

Hezel, D. M., & Simpson, H. B. (2019). Exposure and response prevention for obsessive-compulsive disorder: a review and new directions. *Indian Journal of Psychiatry, 61*(Suppl 1), S85–S92.

Hiç, C., Pradhan, P., Rybski, D., & Kropp, J. P. (2016). Food surplus and its climate burdens. *Environmental Science & Technology, 50*(8), 4269–4277.

HLPE (2017). Nutrition and food systems. *A Report by the High Level Panel of Experts on Food Security and Nutrition of the Committee on World Food Security.* Rome.

Horovitz, O., & Argyrides, M. (2023). Orthorexia and orthorexia nervosa: a comprehensive examination of prevalence, risk factors, diagnosis, and treatment. *Nutrients, 15*(17), 3851.

Howard, C. E., & Porzelius, L. K. (1999). The role of dieting in binge eating disorder: etiology and treatment implications. *Clinical Psychology Review, 19*(1), 25–44.

Hu, F. B. (2002). Dietary pattern analysis: a new direction in nutritional epidemiology. *Current Opinion in Lipidology*, *13*(1), 3–9.

Huynh, P. A., Miles, S., de Boer, K., Meyer, D., & Nedeljkovic, M. (2023). A systematic review and meta-analysis of the relationship between obsessive-compulsive symptoms and symptoms of proposed orthorexia nervosa: the contribution of assessments. *European Eating Disorders Review*, 10.1002/erv.3041. Advance online publication.

Jain, A., & Sharma, U. (2021). Prevalence and relationship of orthorexia nervosa with self-esteem and lifestyle satisfaction in Indian married women. *International Journal of Indian Psychology*, *9*(3), 181–193.

Jordan, C. H., Wang, W., Donatoni, L., & Meier, B. P. (2014). Mindful eating: Trait and state mindfulness predict healthier eating behavior. *Personality and Individual Differences*, *68*, 107–111.

Kalika, E., Egan, H., & Mantzios, M. (2022). Exploring the role of mindful eating and self-compassion on eating behaviours and orthorexia in people following a vegan diet. *Eating and Weight Disorders*, *27*(7), 2641–2651.

Kalika, E., Hussain, M., Egan, H., & Mantzios, M. (2023). Exploring the moderating role of mindfulness, mindful eating, and self-compassion on the relationship between eating-disordered quality of life and orthorexia nervosa. *Eating and Weight Disorders*, *28*(1), 18.

Kaya, S., Uzdil, Z., & Çakıroğlu, F. P. (2022). Validation of the Turkish version of the Orthorexia Nervosa Inventory (ONI) in an adult population: its association with psychometric properties. *Eating and Weight Disorders*, *27*(2), 729–735.

Kessler, U., Kleppe, M. M., Rekkedal, G. Å., Rø, Ø., & Danielsen, Y. (2022). Experiences when implementing enhanced cognitive behavioral therapy as a standard treatment for anorexia nervosa in outpatients at a public specialized eating-disorder treatment unit. *Journal of Eating Disorders*, *10*(1), 15.

Khalil, J., Boutros, S., Kheir, N., Kassem, M., Salameh, P., Sacre, H., Akel, M., Obeid, S., & Hallit, S. (2022). Eating disorders and their relationship with menopausal phases among a sample of middle-aged Lebanese women. *BMC Women's Health*, *22*(1), 153.

King, E., & Wengreen, H. J. (2023). Associations between level of interest in nutrition, knowledge of nutrition, and prevalence of orthorexia traits among undergraduate students. *Nutrition and Health*, *29*(1), 149–155.

Kinzl, J. F., Hauer, K., Traweger, C., & Kiefer, I. (2006). Orthorexia nervosa in dieticians. *Psychotherapy and Psychosomatics*, *75*(6), 395–396.

Kiss-Leizer, M., & Rigó, A. (2019). People behind unhealthy obsession to healthy food: the personality profile of tendency to orthorexia nervosa. *Eating and Weight Disorders*, *24*(1), 29–35.

Kiss-Leizer, M., Tóth-Király, I., & Rigó, A. (2019). How the obsession to eat healthy food meets with the willingness to do sports: the motivational background of orthorexia nervosa. *Eating and Weight Disorders, 24*(3), 465–472.

Knowles, K. A., & Olatunji, B. O. (2023). Intolerance of uncertainty as a cognitive vulnerability for obsessive-compulsive disorder: a qualitative review. *Clinical Psychology: Science and Practice, 30*(3), 317–330.

Kobori, O., Salkovskis, P. M., Read, J., Lounes, N., & Wong, V. (2012). A qualitative study of the investigation of reassurance seeking in obsessive–compulsive disorder. *Journal of Obsessive-Compulsive and Related Disorders, 1*(1), 25–32.

Kok, R. (2020). Emotion regulation. In: Zeigler-Hill, V., & Shackelford, T.K. (Eds.), *Encyclopedia of Personality and Individual Differences.* Cham: Springer.

Koritar, P., & Alvarenga, M. dos S. (2017). Fatores relevantes para uma alimentacao saudavel e para estar saudavel na perspectiva de estudantes de Nutricao [Relevant factors to healthy eating and to be healthy from the perspective of nutrition students]. *Demetra: Food, Nutrition & Health, 12*(4), 1031–1051.

Kouritas, V. K., Papagiannopoulos, K., Lazaridis, G., Baka, S., Mpoukovinas, I., Karavasilis, V., Lampaki, S., Kioumis, I., Pitsiou, G., Papaiwannou, A., Karavergou, A., Kipourou, M., Lada, M., Organtzis, J., Katsikogiannis, N., Tsakiridis, K., Zarogoulidis, K., & Zarogoulidis, P. (2015). Pneumomediastinum. *Journal of Thoracic Disease, 7*(Suppl 1), S44–S49.

Koven, N. S., & Abry, A. W. (2015). The clinical basis of orthorexia nervosa: emerging perspectives. *Neuropsychiatric Disease and Treatment, 11*, 385–394.

Koven, N., & Senbonmatsu, R. (2013) A neuropsychological evaluation of orthorexia nervosa. *Open Journal of Psychiatry, 3*, 214–222.

Krauss, S., Dapp, L. C., & Orth, U. (2023). The link between low self-esteem and eating disorders: a meta-analysis of longitudinal studies. *Clinical Psychological Science, 11*(6), 1141–115.

Kukull, W. A., & Ganguli, M. (2012). Generalizability: the trees, the forest, and the low-hanging fruit. *Neurology, 78*(23), 1886–1891.

Lacroix, E., Tavares, H., & von Ranson, K. M. (2018). Moving beyond the 'eating addiction' versus 'food addiction' debate: comment on Schulte et al. (2017). *Appetite, 130*, 286–292.

Lakritz, C., Tournayre, L., Ouellet, M., Iceta, S., Duriez, P., Masetti, V., & Lafraire, J. (2022). Sinful foods: measuring implicit associations between food categories and moral attributes in anorexic, orthorexic, and healthy subjects. *Frontiers in Nutrition, 9*, 884003.

Lampard, A. M., Tasca, G. A., Balfour, L., & Bissada, H. (2013). An evaluation of the transdiagnostic cognitive-behavioural model of eating disorders. *European Eating Disorders Review, 21*(2), 99–107.

LaSalle, V. H., Cromer, K. R., Nelson, K. N., Kazuba, D., Justement, L., & Murphy, D. L. (2004). Diagnostic interview assessed neuropsychiatric disorder comorbidity in 334 individuals with obsessive-compulsive disorder. *Depression and Anxiety, 19*(3), 163–173.

Lasson, C., Barthels, F., & Raynal, P. (2021). Psychometric evaluation of the French version of the Düsseldorfer Orthorexia Skala (DOS) and prevalence of orthorexia nervosa among university students. *Eating and Weight Disorders, 26*(8), 2589–2596.

Lasson, C., & Raynal, P. (2021). Personality profiles in young adults with orthorexic eating behaviors. *Eating and Weight Disorders, 26*(8), 2727–2736.

Lasson, C., Rousseau, A., Vicente, S., Goutaudier, N., Romo, L., Roncero, M., & Barrada, J. R. (2023). Orthorexic eating behaviors are not all pathological: a French validation of the Teruel Orthorexia Scale (TOS). *Journal of Eating Disorders, 11*(1), 65.

Latiff, A. A., Muhamad, J., & Rahman, R. A. (2018). Body image dissatisfaction and its determinants among young primary-school adolescents. *Journal of Taibah University Medical Sciences, 13*(1), 34–41.

Lee, S. M., Hong, M., Park, S., Kang, W. S., & Oh, I. H. (2021). Economic burden of eating disorders in South Korea. *Journal of Eating Disorders, 9*(1), 30

Lee, R. S. C., Hoppenbrouwers, S., & Franken, I. (2019). A systematic meta-review of impulsivity and compulsivity in addictive behaviors. *Neuropsychology Review, 29*(1), 14–26.

Leppanen, J., Brown, D., McLinden, H., Williams, S., & Tchanturia, K. (2022). The role of emotion regulation in eating disorders: a network meta-analysis approach. *Frontiers in Psychiatry, 13*, 793094.

Lester, H., Tritter, J. Q., & Sorohan, H. (2005). Patients' and health professionals' views on primary care for people with serious mental illness: focus group study. *BMJ, 330*(7500), 1122.

Levin, R. L., Mills, J. S., McComb, S. E., & Rawana, J. S. (2023). Examining orthorexia nervosa: using latent profile analysis to explore potential diagnostic classification and subtypes in a non-clinical sample. *Appetite, 181*, 106398.

Levinson, C.A., Brosof, L.C., Vanzhula, I., Christian, C., Jones, P., Rodebaugh, T.L., Langer, J.K., White, E.K., Warren, C., Weeks, J.W., et al. (2018). Social anxiety and eating disorder comorbidity and underlying vulnerabilities: using network analysis to conceptualize comorbidity. *International Journal of Eating Disorders, 51*, 693–709.

Lewthwaite, M., & LaMarre, A. (2022). 'That's just healthy eating in my opinion' – balancing understandings of health and 'orthorexic' dietary and exercise practices. *Appetite*, *171*, 105938.

Li, W. L., Tan, S. X., Ouyang, R. Q., Cui, Y. F., Ma, J. R., Cheng, C., Mu, Y. J., Zhang, S. W., Zheng, L., Xiong, P., Ni, W. Z., Li, L. Y., Fan, L. N., Luo, Y. M., Yu, Y. L., Wang, Z. M., Ding, F., Pan, Q. F., Jiang, A. Y., Huang, J. M., … Zeng, F. F. (2022). Translation and validation of the Chinese version of the orthorexia nervosa assessment questionnaires among college students. *Eating and Weight Disorders*, *27*(8), 3389–3398.

Liddell, H.G., & Scott, R. (1996). *Greek-English Lexicon*. Oxford University Press.

Limburg, K., Watson, H. J., Hagger, M. S., & Egan, S. J. (2017). The relationship between perfectionism and psychopathology: a meta-analysis. *Journal of Clinical Psychology*, *73*(10), 1301–1326.

Lobstein, T. & Davies, S. 2008. Defining and labelling 'healthy' and 'unhealthy' food. *Public Health Nutrition*, *12*(3), 331–340.

Lopes, R., Melo, R., & Dias Pereira, B. (2020). Orthorexia nervosa and comorbid depression successfully treated with mirtazapine: a case report. *Eating and Weight Disorders*, *25*(1), 163–167.

López-Gil, J. F., Tárraga-López, P. J., Hershey, M. S., López-Bueno, R., Gutiérrez-Espinoza, H., Soler Marín, A., Fernández-Montero, A., & Victoria-Montesinos, D. (2023). Overall proportion of orthorexia nervosa symptoms: a systematic review and meta-analysis including 30,476 individuals from 18 countries. *Journal of Global Health*, *13*, 04087.

Luck-Sikorski, C., Jung, F., Schlosser, K., & Riedel-Heller, S. G. (2019). Is orthorexic behavior common in the general public? A large representative study in Germany. *Eating and Weight Disorders*, *24*(2), 267–273.

Luo, M., & Allman-Farinelli, M. (2021). Trends in the number of behavioural theory-based healthy eating interventions inclusive of dietitians/nutritionists in 2000–2020. *Nutrients*, *13*(11), 4161.

Luo, X., Donnellan, M. B., Burt, S. A., & Klump, K. L. (2016). The dimensional nature of eating pathology: evidence from a direct comparison of categorical, dimensional, and hybrid models. *Journal of Abnormal Psychology*, *125*(5), 715–726.

MacDuff, A., Arnold, A., Harvey, J., & BTS Pleural Disease Guideline Group (2010). Management of spontaneous pneumothorax: British Thoracic Society Pleural Disease Guideline 2010. *Thorax*, *65*(suppl 2), ii18–ii31.

Mahfoud, D., Pardini, S., Mróz, M., Hallit, S., Obeid, S., Akel, M., Novara, C., & Brytek-Matera, A. (2023). Profiling orthorexia nervosa in young adults: the role of obsessive behaviour, perfectionism, and self-esteem. *Journal of Eating Disorders*, *11*(1), 188.

Maïano, C., Aimé, A., Almenara, C. A., Gagnon, C., & Barrada, J. R. (2022). Psychometric properties of the Teruel Orthorexia Scale (TOS) among a French-Canadian adult sample. *Eating and Weight Disorders*, *27*(8), 3457–3467.

Malhi, G. S., Bell, E., Bassett, D., Boyce, P., Bryant, R., Hazell, P., Hopwood, M., Lyndon, B., Mulder, R., Porter, R., Singh, A. B., & Murray, G. (2021). The 2020 Royal Australian and New Zealand College of Psychiatrists clinical practice guidelines for mood disorders. *Australian and New Zealand Journal of Psychiatry*, *55*(1), 7–117.

Malmborg, J., Bremander, A., Olsson, M. C., & Bergman, S. (2017). Health status, physical activity, and orthorexia nervosa: a comparison between exercise science students and business students. *Appetite*, *109*, 137–143.

Mantzios M. (2021). (Re)defining mindful eating into mindful eating behaviour to advance scientific enquiry. *Nutrition and Health*, *27*(4), 367–371.

Mantzios, M., Egan, H., Hussain, M., Keyte, R., & Bahia, H. (2018). Mindfulness, self-compassion, and mindful eating in relation to fat and sugar consumption: an exploratory investigation. *Eating and Weight Disorders*, *23*(6), 833–840.

Mantzios, M., Skillett, K., & Egan, H. (2019). Examining the effects of two mindful eating exercises on chocolate consumption: an experimental study. *European Journal of Health Psychology*, *26*(4), 120–128.

Martinovic, D., Tokic, D., Martinovic, L., Vilovic, M., Vrdoljak, J., Kumric, M., Bukic, J., Ticinovic Kurir, T., Tavra, M., & Bozic, J. (2022). Adherence to Mediterranean diet and tendency to orthorexia nervosa in professional athletes. *Nutrients*, *14*(2), 237.

Martins, M. C. T., Alvarenga, M. dos S., Vargas, S. V. A., Sato, K. S. C. de J., & Scagliusi, F. B. (2011). Ortorexia nervosa: reflexões sobre um novo conceito. *Revista de Nutrição*, *24*(2), 345–357.

Mattei, J., & Alfonso, C. (2020). Strategies for healthy eating promotion and behavioral change perceived as effective by nutrition professionals: a mixed-methods study. *Frontiers in Nutrition*, *7*, 114.

Mathieu J. (2005). What is orthorexia?. *Journal of the American Dietetic Association*, *105*(10), 1510–1512.

Mavrandrea, P., & Gonidakis, F. (2023). Exercise dependence and orthorexia nervosa in Crossfit: exploring the role of perfectionism. *Current Psychology*, *42*, 25151–25159.

Mavrović, J. B. (2023). Development of eating disorders in the socio-historical context. In J. Balabanić Mavrović (Ed.), *Eating Disorders in a Capitalist World: Super Woman or a Super Failure?* (pp. 23–40). Emerald Publishing Limited.

McComb, S. E., & Mills, J. S. (2019). Orthorexia nervosa: a review of psychosocial risk factors. *Appetite, 140*, 50–75.

McDonald, A., & Braun V. (2022). Right, yet impossible? Constructions of healthy eating. *SSM – Qualitative Research in Health, 2*, 100100.

McGovern, L., Gaffney, M., & Trimble, T. (2021). The experience of orthorexia from the perspective of recovered orthorexics. *Eating and Weight Disorders, 26*(5), 1375–1388.

McLean, C. P., Kulkarni, J., & Sharp, G. (2022). Disordered eating and the meat-avoidance spectrum: a systematic review and clinical implications. *Eating and Weight Disorders, 27*(7), 2347–2375.

Meier, M., Kossakowski, J. J., Jones, P. J., Kay, B., Riemann, B. C., & McNally, R. J. (2020). Obsessive-compulsive symptoms in eating disorders: a network investigation. *International Journal of Eating Disorders, 53*(3), 362–371.

Melhorn, J., & Davies, H.E. (2021). The management of subcutaneous emphysema in pneumothorax: a literature review *Current Pulmonology Reports, 10*, 92–97.

Melina, V., Craig, W., & Levin, S. (2016). Position of the Academy of Nutrition and Dietetics: vegetarian diets. *Journal of the Academy of Nutrition and Dietetics, 116*(12), 1970–1980.

Merhy, G., Moubarak, V., Hallit, R., Obeid, S., & Hallit, S. (2023). The indirect role of orthorexia nervosa and eating attitudes in the association between perfectionism and muscle dysmorphic disorder in Lebanese male University students – results of a pilot study. *BMC Psychiatry, 23*(1), 55.

Messer, M., Liu, C., & Linardon, J. (2023). Orthorexia nervosa symptoms prospectively predict symptoms of eating disorders and depression. *Eating Behaviors, 49*, 101734.

Messer, M., Liu, C., McClure, Z., Mond, J., Tiffin, C., & Linardon, J. (2022). Negative body image components as risk factors for orthorexia nervosa: prospective findings. *Appetite, 178*, 106280.

Meule, A., Holzapfel, C., Brandl, B., Greetfeld, M., Hessler-Kaufmann, J. B., Skurk, T., Quadflieg, N., Schlegl, S., Hauner, H., & Voderholzer, U. (2020). Measuring orthorexia nervosa: a comparison of four self-report questionnaires. *Appetite, 146*, 104512.

Meule, A., & Voderholzer, U. (2021). Orthorexia nervosa – it is time to think about abandoning the concept of a distinct diagnosis. *Frontiers in Psychiatry, 12*, 640401.

Mhanna, M., Azzi, R., Hallit, S., Obeid, S., & Soufia, M. (2022). Validation of the Arabic version of the Teruel Orthorexia Scale (TOS) among Lebanese adolescents. *Eating and Weight Disorders, 27*(2), 619–627.

Micali, N., Martini, M. G., Thomas, J. J., Eddy, K. T., Kothari, R., Russell, E., Bulik, C. M., & Treasure, J. (2017). Lifetime and 12-month prevalence of eating disorders amongst women in mid-life: a population-based study of diagnoses and risk factors. *BMC Medicine, 15*(1), 12.

Miley, M., Egan, H., Wallis, D., & Mantzios, M. (2022). Orthorexia nervosa, mindful eating, and perfectionism: an exploratory investigation. *Eating and Weight Disorders, 27*(7), 2869–2878.

Missbach, B., Dunn, T. M., & König, J. S. (2017). We need new tools to assess orthorexia nervosa. A commentary on 'Prevalence of orthorexia nervosa among college students based on Bratman's Test and associated tendencies'. *Appetite, 108*, 521–524.

Missbach, B., Hinterbuchinger, B., Dreiseitl, V., Zellhofer, S., Kurz, C., & König, J. (2015). When eating right, is measured wrong! A validation and critical examination of the ORTO-15 questionnaire in German. *PloS One, 10*(8), e0135772.

Mitrofanova, E., Pummell, E., Martinelli, L., & Petróczi, A. (2021). Does ORTO-15 produce valid data for 'Orthorexia Nervosa'? A mixed-method examination of participants' interpretations of the fifteen test items. *Eating and Weight Disorders, 26*(3), 897–909.

Mohamed Halim, Z., Dickinson, K. M., Kemps, E., & Prichard, I. (2020). Orthorexia nervosa: examining the Eating Habits Questionnaire's reliability and validity, and its links to dietary adequacy among adult women. *Public Health Nutrition, 23*(10), 1684–1692.

Molendijk, M., Molero, P., Ortuño Sánchez-Pedreño, F., Van der Does, W., & Angel Martínez-González, M. (2018). Diet quality and depression risk: a systematic review and dose-response meta-analysis of prospective studies. *Journal of Affective Disorders, 226*, 346–354.

Moller, S., Apputhurai, P., & Knowles, S. R. (2019). Confirmatory factor analyses of the ORTO 15-, 11- and 9-item scales and recommendations for suggested cut-off scores. *Eating and Weight Disorders : EWD, 24*(1), 21–28.

Monterrosa, E. C., Frongillo, E. A., Drewnowski, A., de Pee, S., & Vandevijvere, S. (2020). Sociocultural influences on food choices and implications for sustainable healthy diets. *Food and Nutrition Bulletin, 41*(2_suppl), 59S–73S.

Moroze, R. M., Dunn, T. M., Craig Holland, J., Yager, J., & Weintraub, P. (2015). Microthinking about micronutrients: a case of transition from obsessions about healthy eating to near-fatal 'orthorexia nervosa' and proposed diagnostic criteria. *Psychosomatics, 56*(4), 397–403.

Mozaffarian, D., & Ludwig, D. S. (2010). Dietary guidelines in the 21st century: a time for food. *JAMA, 304*(6), 681–682.

Murphy, R., Nutzinger, D. O., Paul, T., & Leplow, B. (2004). Conditional-associative learning in eating disorders: a comparison with OCD. *Journal of Clinical and Experimental Neuropsychology, 26*(2), 190–199.

Murphy, R., Straebler, S., Cooper, Z., & Fairburn, C. G. (2010). Cognitive behavioral therapy for eating disorders. *Psychiatric Clinics of North America, 33*(3), 611–627.

Musolino, C., Warin, M., Wade, T., & Gilchrist, P. (2015). 'Healthy anorexia': the complexity of care in disordered eating. *Social Science & Medicine, 139*, 18–25.

Nadel, I. B. (1982). Moments in the Greenwood: *Maurice* in context. In: Herz, J.S., & Martin, R.K. (Eds.), *Centenary Revaluations* (pp. 177–190). London: Palgrave Macmillan.

National Health Service (2022). *Eating a Balanced Diet*. www.nhs.uk/live-well/eat-well/how-to-eat-a-balanced-diet/eating-a-balanced-diet/

National Institute for Health and Care Excellence (NICE, 2017). *Eating Disorders: Recognition and Treatment*. NICE Guideline 69, London: NICE.

Navarro, A., Varela, C., Fusté, A., Andrés, A., & Saldaña, C. (2023). The validation of the Barcelona Orthorexia Scale-Spanish version: evidence from the general population. *Eating and Weight Disorders, 28*(1), 90.

Nazareth, M., Richards, J., Javalkar, K., Haberman, C., Zhong, Y., Rak, E., Jain, N., Ferris, M., & van Tilburg, M. A. (2016). Relating health locus of control to health care use, adherence, and transition readiness among youths with chronic conditions, North Carolina, 2015. *Preventing Chronic Disease, 13*, E93.

Nelson, J. B. (2017). Mindful eating: the art of presence while you eat. *Diabetes, 30*(3), 171–174.

Neumark-Sztainer, D., Wall, M., Larson, N. I., Eisenberg, M. E., & Loth, K. (2011). Dieting and disordered eating behaviors from adolescence to young adulthood: findings from a 10-year longitudinal study. *Journal of the American Dietetic Association, 111*(7), 1004–1011.

Nezgovorova, V., Reid, J., Fineberg, N. A., & Hollander, E. (2022). Optimizing first line treatments for adults with OCD. *Comprehensive Psychiatry, 115*, 152305.

Ng, L. W., Ng, D. P., & Wong, W. P. (2013). Is supervised exercise training safe in patients with anorexia nervosa? A meta-analysis. *Physiotherapy, 99*(1), 1–11.

Niedzielski, A., & Kaźmierczak-Wojtaś, N. (2021). Prevalence of orthorexia nervosa and its diagnostic tools: a Literature Review. *International Journal of Environmental Research and Public Health, 18*(10), 5488.

Norris, M. L., Spettigue, W., Hammond, N. G., Katzman, D. K., Zucker, N., Yelle, K., … & Obeid, N. (2018). Building evidence for the use of descriptive subtypes in youth with avoidant restrictive food intake disorder. *International Journal of Eating Disorders*, *51*(2), 170–173.

Novara, C., Maggio, E., Piasentin, S., Pardini, S., & Mattioli, S. (2021a). Orthorexia nervosa: differences between clinical and non-clinical samples. *BMC Psychiatry*, *21*(1), 341.

Novara, C., Mattioli, S., Piasentin, S., Pardini, S., & Maggio, E. (2022a). The role of dieting, psychopathological characteristics and maladaptive personality traits in orthorexia nervosa. *BMC Psychiatry*, *22*(1), 290.

Novara, C., Pardini, S., Maggio, E., Mattioli, S., & Piasentin, S. (2021b). Orthorexia nervosa: over concern or obsession about healthy food? *Eating and Weight Disorders*, *26*(8), 2577–2588.

Novara, C., Piasentin, S., Mattioli, S., Pardini, S., & Maggio, E. (2023). Perfectionism or perfectionisms in orthorexia nervosa. *Nutrients*, *15*(15), 3289.

Novara, C., Pardini, S., Visioli, F., & Meda, N. (2022b). Orthorexia nervosa and dieting in a non-clinical sample: a prospective study. *Eating and Weight Disorders*, *27*(6), 2081–2093.

Nyman H. (2002). En rak fråga: ortorexi rätt ord på fel sak? [A direct question: is orthorexia a correct word for a wrong concept?]. *Lakartidningen*, *99*(5), 423–424.

Obara, A. A., Vivolo, S. R. G. F., & Alvarenga, M. dos S. (2018). Weight bias in nutritional practice: a study with nutrition students. Preconceito relacionado ao peso na conduta nutricional: um estudo com estudantes de nutrição. *Cadernos de Saude Publica*, *34*(8), e00088017.

Obeid, S., Hallit, S., Akel, M., & Brytek-Matera, A. (2021). Orthorexia nervosa and its association with alexithymia, emotion dysregulation and disordered eating attitudes among Lebanese adults. *Eating and Weight Disorders*, *26*(8), 2607–2616.

Oberle, C. D., De Nadai, A. S., & Madrid, A. L. (2021). Orthorexia Nervosa Inventory (ONI): development and validation of a new measure of orthorexic symptomatology. *Eating and Weight Disorders*, *26*(2), 609–622.

Oberle, C. D., Klare, D. L., & Patyk, K. C. (2019). Health beliefs, behaviors, and symptoms associated with orthorexia nervosa. *Eating and Weight Disorders*, *24*(3), 495–506.

Oberle, C. D., & Lipschuetz, S. L. (2018). Orthorexia symptoms correlate with perceived muscularity and body fat, not BMI. *Eating and Weight Disorders*, *23*(3), 363–368.

Oberle, C. D., & Noebel, N.A. (2023). Assessment of orthorexia nervosa. In: A. Meule (Ed.). *Assessment of Eating Behavior* (pp. 56–70). Göttingen, Germany: Hogrefe.

Oberle, C. D., Samaghabadi, R. O., & Hughes, E. M. (2017). Orthorexia nervosa: Assessment and correlates with gender, BMI, and personality. *Appetite, 108,* 303–310.

Oberle, C. D., Watkins, R. S., & Burkot, A. J. (2018). Orthorexic eating behaviors related to exercise addiction and internal motivations in a sample of university students. *Eating and Weight Disorders, 23*(1), 67–74.

Opitz, M. C., Newman, E., Alvarado Vázquez Mellado, A. S., Robertson, M. D. A., & Sharpe, H. (2020). The psychometric properties of Orthorexia Nervosa assessment scales: a systematic review and reliability generalization. *Appetite, 155,* 104797.

Opitz, M-C., Newman, E., & Sharpe, H. (2022). Understanding perceived characteristics and causes of orthorexia nervosa in online communities: a Reddit analysis. *Cyberpsychology: Journal of Psychosocial Research on Cyberspace, 16*(5), Article 6.

Orlinski, D. E., Grawe, E., & Parks, B. K. (1994). Process and outcome in psychotherapy: noch einmal. In A. E. Garfield, & S. L. Garfield (Eds.), *Handbook of Psychotherapy and Behaviour Change* (4th edition, pp. 270–378). New York: Wiley.

Özdengül, F., Yargic, M. P., Solak, R., Yaylali, O., & Kurklu, G. B. (2021). Assessment of orthorexia nervosa via ORTO-R scores of Turkish recreational and competitive athletes and sedentary individuals: a cross-sectional questionnaire study. *Eating and Weight Disorders, 26*(4), 1111–1118.

Özenoğlu, A., & Ünal, G. (2015). The effect of self-esteem and incidence of orthorexia nervosa among university students of health education. *Journal of International Research in Medical and Pharmaceutical Sciences, 6*(4), 173–182.

Paludo, A. C., Gimunová, M., Michaelides, M., Kobus, M., & Parpa, K. (2023). Description of the menstrual cycle status, energy availability, eating behavior and physical performance in a youth female soccer team. *Scientific Reports, 13*(1), 11194.

Paludo, A. C., Magatão, M., Martins, H. R. F., Martins, M. V. S., & Kumstát, M. (2022). Prevalence of risk for orthorexia in athletes using the ORTO-15 Questionnaire: A systematic mini-review. *Frontiers in Psychology, 13,* 856185.

Park, S. W., Kim, J. Y., Go, G. J., Jeon, E. S., Pyo, H. J., & Kwon, Y. J. (2011). Orthorexia nervosa with hyponatremia, subcutaneous emphysema, pneumomediastimum, pneumothorax, and pancytopenia. *Electrolyte & Blood Pressure, 9*(1), 32–37.

Parra-Fernández, M. L., Manzaneque-Cañadillas, M., Onieva-Zafra, M. D., Fernández-Martínez, E., Fernández-Muñoz, J. J., Prado-Laguna, M. D. C., & Brytek-Matera, A. (2020). Pathological preoccupation with healthy eating (orthorexia nervosa) in a Spanish sample with vegetarian, vegan, and non-vegetarian dietary patterns. *Nutrients, 12*(12), 3907.

Parra-Fernández, M. L., Onieva-Zafra, M. D., Fernández-Muñoz, J. J., & Fernández-Martínez, E. (2019). Adaptation and validation of the Spanish version of the DOS questionnaire for the detection of orthorexic nervosa behavior. *PloS One, 14*(5), e0216583.

Parra-Fernández, M. L., Onieva-Zafra, M. D., Fernández-Muñoz, J. J., Głębocka, A., Fernández-Martínez, E., & Brytek-Matera, A. (2021). The Spanish version of the Eating Habits Questionnaire (EHQ-ES) and its links to symptoms and concerns characteristic of eating disorders among young adults. *Nutrients, 13*(6), 1993.

Parra-Fernández, M. L., Rodríguez-Cano, T., Onieva-Zafra, M. D., Perez-Haro, M. J., Casero-Alonso, V., Fernández-Martínez, E., & Notario-Pacheco, B. (2018a). Prevalence of orthorexia nervosa in university students and its relationship with psychopathological aspects of eating behaviour disorders. *BMC Psychiatry, 18*(1), 364.

Parra-Fernández, M. L., Rodríguez-Cano, T., Onieva-Zafra, M. D., Perez-Haro, M. J., Casero-Alonso, V., Muñoz Camargo, J. C., & Notario-Pacheco, B. (2018b). Adaptation and validation of the Spanish version of the ORTO-15 questionnaire for the diagnosis of orthorexia nervosa. *PloS One, 13*(1), e0190722.

Pauligk, S., Seidel, M., Fürtjes, S., King, J. A., Geisler, D., Hellerhoff, I., Roessner, V., Schmidt, U., Goschke, T., Walter, H., Strobel, A., & Ehrlich, S. (2021). The costs of over-control in anorexia nervosa: evidence from fMRI and ecological momentary assessment. *Translational Psychiatry, 11*(1), 304.

Pauzé, A., Plouffe-Demers, M. P., Fiset, D., Saint-Amour, D., Cyr, C., & Blais, C. (2021). The relationship between orthorexia nervosa symptomatology and body image attitudes and distortion. *Scientific Reports, 11*(1), 13311.

Pinto, A., Mancebo, M. C., Eisen, J. L., Pagano, M. E., & Rasmussen, S. A. (2006). The Brown Longitudinal Obsessive Compulsive Study: clinical features and symptoms of the sample at intake. *Journal of Clinical Psychiatry, 67*(5), 703–711.

Plichta, M., & Jeżewska-Zychowicz, M. (2019). Eating behaviors, attitudes toward health and eating, and symptoms of orthorexia nervosa among students. *Appetite, 137*, 114–123.

Plichta, M., Jeżewska-Zychowicz, M., & Gębski, J. (2019). Orthorexic tendency in Polish students: exploring association with dietary patterns, body satisfaction and weight. *Nutrients, 11*(1), 100.

Polit, D. F., & Beck, C. T. (2010). Generalization in quantitative and qualitative research: myths and strategies. *International Journal of Nursing Studies*, *47*(11), 1451–1458.

Polivy, J., & Herman, C. P. (1985). Dieting and binging: a causal analysis. *American Psychologist*, *40*(2), 193–201.

Poyraz, C. A., Tüfekçioğlu, E. Y., Özdemir, A., Baş, A., Kani, A. S., Erginöz, E., & Duran, A. (2015). Relationship between orthorexia and obsessive-compulsive symptoms in patients with generalised anxiety disorder, panic disorder and obsessive-compulsive disorder. *Neuropsychiatric Investigation*, *53*(4), 22–26.

Prestwich, A., Sniehotta, F. F., Whittington, C., Dombrowski, S. U., Rogers, L., & Michie, S. (2014). Does theory influence the effectiveness of health behavior interventions? Meta-analysis. *Health Psychology*, *33*(5), 465–474.

Public Health England (2016a). *The Eatwell Guide*. Public Health England in association with the Welsh Government FSSatFSAiNI. Contract No.: 9 August 2016.

Public Health England (2016b). *From Plate to Guide: What, Why and How for the Eatwell Model*. https://assets.publishing.service.gov.uk/media/5a7f-73f7e5274a2e8ab4c461/eatwell_model_guide_report.pdf.

Radomsky A. S. (2022). The fear of losing control. *Journal of Behavior Therapy and Experimental Psychiatry*, *77*, 101768.

Raine K. D. (2005). Determinants of healthy eating in Canada: an overview and synthesis. *Canadian Journal of Public Health (Revue Canadienne de Santé Publique)*, *96* Suppl 3(Suppl 3), S8–S15.

Rania, M., de Filippis, R., Caroleo, M., Carbone, E., Aloi, M., Bratman, S., & Segura-Garcia, C. (2021). Pathways to orthorexia nervosa: a case series discussion. *Eating and Weight Disorders*, *26*(5), 1675–1683.

Raynal, P., Soccodato, M., Fages, M., & Séjourné, N. (2022). A comparative study of orthorexia between premenopausal, perimenopausal, and postmenopausal women. *Eating and Weight Disorders*, *27*(7), 2523–2531.

Reilly, E. E., Brown, T. A., Gray, E. K., Kaye, W. H., & Menzel, J. E. (2019). Exploring the cooccurrence of behavioural phenotypes for avoidant/restrictive food intake disorder in a partial hospitalization sample. *European Eating Disorders Review*, *27*(4), 429–435.

Reinstein, N., Koszewski, W. M., Chamberlin, B., & Smith-Johnson, C. (1992). Prevalence of eating disorders among dietetics students: does nutrition education make a difference? *Journal of the American Dietetic Association*, *92*(8), 949–953.

Reuven-Magril, O., Dar, R., & Liberman, N. (2008). Illusion of control and behavioral control attempts in obsessive-compulsive disorder. *Journal of Abnormal Psychology*, *117*(2), 334–341.

Reynolds R. (2018). Is the prevalence of orthorexia nervosa in an Australian university population 6.5%? *Eating and Weight Disorders, 23*(4), 453–458.

Reynolds, R., McGowan, A., Smith, S., & Rawstorne, P. (2023). Vegan and vegetarian males and females have higher orthorexic traits than omnivores, and are motivated in their food choice by factors including ethics and weight control. *Nutrition and Health,* 2601060231187924. Advance online publication.

Reynolds, R., & McMahon, S. (2019). Views of health professionals on the clinical recognition of orthorexia nervosa: a pilot study. *Eating and Weight Disorders, 25*, 1117–1124.

Rigby, R. R., Mitchell, L. J., Hamilton, K., & Williams, L. T. (2020). The use of behavior change theories in dietetics practice in primary health care: a systematic review of randomized controlled trials. *Journal of the Academy of Nutrition and Dietetics, 120*(7), 1172–1197.

Ringwald, W. R., Forbes, M. K., & Wright, A. G. (2023). Meta-analysis of structural evidence for the Hierarchical Taxonomy of Psychopathology (HiTOP) model. *Psychological Medicine, 53*(2), 533–546.

Roberto da Silva, W., Cruz Marmol, C. H., Nogueira Neves, A., Marôco, J., & Bonini Campos, J. A. D. (2021). A Portuguese adaptation of the Teruel Orthorexia Scale and a test of its utility with Brazilian young adults. *Perceptual and Motor Skills, 128*(5), 2052–2074.

Robins, E., & Guze, S. B. (1970). Establishment of diagnostic validity in psychiatric illness: its application to schizophrenia. *American Journal of Psychiatry, 126*(7), 983–987.

Robinson, K. A., Brunnhuber, K., Ciliska, D., Juhl, C. B., Christensen, R., Lund, H., & Evidence-Based Research Network (2021). Evidence-Based Research Series – paper 1: what evidence-based research is and why is it important? *Journal of Clinical Epidemiology, 129*, 151–157.

Rodebaugh, T. L., Scullin, R. B., Langer, J. K., Dixon, D. J., Huppert, J. D., Bernstein, A., Zvielli, A., & Lenze, E. J. (2016). Unreliability as a threat to understanding psychopathology: the cautionary tale of attentional bias. *Journal of Abnormal Psychology, 125*(6), 840–851.

Rodgers, R. F., White, M., & Berry, R. (2021). Orthorexia nervosa, intuitive eating, and eating competence in female and male college students. *Eating and Weight Disorders, 26*(8), 2625–2632.

Rogowska, A. M., Kwaśnicka, A., & Ochnik, D. (2021). Development and validation of the Test of Orthorexia Nervosa (TON-17). *Journal of Clinical Medicine, 10*(8), 1637.

Rogoza, R., & Donini, L. M. (2021). Introducing ORTO-R: a revision of ORTO-15: based on the re-assessment of original data. *Eating and Weight Disorders, 26*(3), 887–895.

Rogoza, R., Hallit, S., Soufia, M., Barthels, F., & Obeid, S. (2021). Validation of the Arabic version of the Dusseldorf Orthorexia Scale (DOS) among Lebanese adolescents. *Journal of Eating Disorders, 9*(1), 130.

Rogoza, R., Mhanna, M., Gerges, S., Donini, L. M., Obeid, S., & Hallit, S. (2022). Validation of the Arabic version of the ORTO-R among a sample of Lebanese young adults. *Eating and Weight Disorders, 27*(6), 2073–2080.

Roncero, M., Barrada, J. R., & Perpiñá, C. (2017). Measuring orthorexia nervosa: psychometric limitations of the ORTO-15. *Spanish Journal of Psychology, 20*, E41.

Roncero, M., Barrada, J. R., García-Soriano, G., & Guillén, V. (2021). Personality profile in orthorexia nervosa and healthy orthorexia. *Frontiers in Psychology, 12*, 710604.

Rosenberg, M. (1965). *Society and the Adolescent Self-Image.* Princeton, NJ: Princeton University Press.

Ross Arguedas, A. A. (2020). 'Can naughty be healthy?': healthism and its discontents in news coverage of orthorexia nervosa. *Social Science & Medicine, 246*, 112784.

Rudolph S. (2018). The connection between exercise addiction and orthorexia nervosa in German fitness sports. *Eating and Weight Disorders, 23*(5), 581–586.

Ryman, F. V. M., Cesuroglu, T., Bood, Z. M., & Syurina, E. V. (2019). Orthorexia nervosa: disorder or not? Opinions of Dutch health professionals. *Frontiers in Psychology, 10*, 555.

Saddichha, S., Babu, G. N., & Chandra, P. (2012). Orthorexia nervosa presenting as prodrome of schizophrenia. *Schizophrenia Research, 134*(1), 110.

Sala, M., Rochefort, C., Lui, P. P., & Baldwin, A. S. (2020). Trait mindfulness and health behaviours: a meta-analysis. *Health Psychology Review, 14*(3), 345–393.

Salmela, J., Konttinen, H., Lappalainen, R., Muotka, J., Antikainen, A., Lindström, J., Tuomilehto, J., Uusitupa, M., & Karhunen, L. (2023). Eating behavior dimensions and 9-year weight loss maintenance: a sub-study of the Finnish diabetes prevention study. *International Journal of Obesity, 47*(7), 564–573.

Samaha, S., Azzi, R., Rizk, R., Sarray El Dine, A., Malaeb, D., Hallit, S., Obeid, S., & Soufia, M. (2022). Association between the bi-dimensional aspect of orthorexia and healthy behaviors among Lebanese adolescents. *BMC Psychiatry, 22*(1), 725.

Sanchez-Cerezo, J., Neale, J., Julius, N., Croudace, T., Lynn, R. M., Hudson, L. D., & Nicholls, D. Subtypes of avoidant/restrictive food intake disorder in children and adolescents: a latent class analysis. *Lancet.* Preprint.

Santarossa, S., Lacasse, J., Larocque, J., & Woodruff, S. J. (2019). #Orthorexia on Instagram: a descriptive study exploring the online conversation and community using the Netlytic software. *Eating and Weight Disorders, 24*(2), 283–290.

Sanzari, C. M., & Hormes, J. M. (2023). U.S. health professionals' perspectives on orthorexia nervosa: clinical utility, measurement and diagnosis, and perceived influence of sociocultural factors. *Eating and Weight Disorders, 28*(1), 31.

Scarff J. R. (2017). Orthorexia nervosa: an obsession with healthy eating. *Federal Practitioner, 34*(6), 36–39.

Sagui-Henson, S. J., Radin, R. M., Jhaveri, K., Brewer, J. A., Cohn, M., Hartogensis, W., & Mason, A. E. (2021). Negative mood and food craving strength among women with overweight: implications for targeting mechanisms using a mindful eating intervention. *Mindfulness, 12*(12), 2997–3010.

Scheiber, R., Diehl, S., & Karmasin, M. (2023). Socio-cultural power of social media on orthorexia nervosa: an empirical investigation on the mediating role of thin-ideal and muscular internalization, appearance comparison, and body dissatisfaction. *Appetite, 185*, 106522.

Seguias, L., & Tapper, K. (2018). The effect of mindful eating on subsequent intake of a high calorie snack. *Appetite, 121*, 93–100.

Segura-Garcia, C., Papaianni, M. C., Caglioti, F., Procopio, L., Nisticò, C. G., Bombardiere, L., Ammendolia, A., Rizza, P., De Fazio, P., & Capranica, L. (2012). Orthorexia nervosa: a frequent eating disordered behavior in athletes. *Eating and Weight Disorders, 17*(4), e226–e233.

Segura-Garcia C., Ramacciotti, C., Rania, M., Aloi, M., Caroleo, M., Bruni, A., Gazzarrini, D., Sinopoli, F., & De Fazio, P. (2015). The prevalence of orthorexia nervosa among eating disorder patients after treatment. *Eating and Weight Disorders, 20*(2), 161–166.

Setnick, J. (2013) *The Eating Disorders Clinical Pocket Guide: Quick reference for Healthcare Providers*, second edition. Dallas: Understanding Nutrition.

Sezer Katar, K., Şahin, B., & Kurtoğlu, M. B. (2023). Healthy orthorexia, orthorexia nervosa, and personality traits in a community sample in Turkey. *International Journal of Psychiatry in Medicine*, 912174231194745. Advance online publication.

Sfeir, M., Malaeb, D., Obeid, S., & Hallit, S. (2022). Association between religiosity and orthorexia nervosa with the mediating role of self-esteem among a sample of the Lebanese population: short communication. *Journal of Eating Disorders, 10*(1), 151.

Shafran, R., Cooper, Z., & Fairburn, C. G. (2002). Clinical perfectionism: a cognitive-behavioural analysis. *Behaviour Research and Therapy*, *40*(7), 773–791.

Shah, S. M. (2012). Orthorexia nervosa: healthy eating or eating disorder? Master's Thesis. https://thekeep.eiu.edu/theses/991.

Short, S. E., & Mollborn, S. (2015). Social determinants and health behaviors: conceptual frames and empirical advances. *Current Opinion in Psychology*, *5*, 78–84.

Simons, C. W. & Hall, C., 3rd. (2017). Consumer acceptability of gluten-free cookies containing raw cooked and germinated pinto bean flours. *Food Science & Nutrition*, *6*(1), 77–84.

Souza, H. M. A. V., do Carmo, A. S., & Dos Santos, L. C. (2021). The Brazilian version of the DOS for the detection of orthorexia nervosa: transcultural adaptation and validation among dietitians and nutrition college students. *Eating and Weight Disorders*, *26*(8), 2713–2725.

Sultana, M. S., Islam, M. S., Sayeed, A., Koly, K. N., Baker, K., Hossain, R., Ahmed, S., Ferdous, M. Z., Mubarak, M., Potenza, M. N., & Sikder, M. T. (2022). Food addiction, orthorexia nervosa and dietary diversity among Bangladeshi university students: a large online survey during the COVID-19 pandemic. *Journal of Eating Disorders*, *10*(1), 163.

Surała, O., Malczewska-Lenczowska, J., Sadowska, D., Grabowska, I., & Białecka-Dębek, A. (2020). Traits of orthorexia nervosa and the determinants of these behaviors in elite athletes. *Nutrients*, *12*(9), 2683.

Statista (2023). www.statista.com/statistics/1380282/daily-time-spent-online-global/.

Staudacher, H. M., & Harer, K. N. (2018). When clean eating goes dirty. *The Lancet. Gastroenterology & Hepatology*, *3*(10), 668.

Sternheim, L., Startup, H., & Schmidt, U. (2011). An experimental exploration of behavioral and cognitive-emotional aspects of intolerance of uncertainty in eating disorder patients. *Journal of Anxiety Disorders*, *25*(6), 806–812.

Strahler J. (2021). Trait mindfulness differentiates the interest in healthy diet from orthorexia nervosa. *Eating and Weight Disorders*, *26*(3), 993–998.

Strahler, J., Hermann, A., Walter, B., & Stark, R. (2018). Orthorexia nervosa: a behavioral complex or a psychological condition? *Journal of Behavioral Addictions*, *7*(4), 1143–1156.

Strahler, J., & Stark, R. (2020). Perspective: classifying orthorexia nervosa as a new mental illness – much discussion, little evidence. *Advances in Nutrition*, *11*(4), 784–789.

Strahler, J., Haddad, C., Salameh, P., Sacre, H., Obeid, S., & Hallit, S. (2020). Cross-cultural differences in orthorexic eating behaviors: associations with personality traits. *Nutrition*, *77*, 110811.

Strahler, J., Wachten, H., & Mueller-Alcazar, A. (2021). Obsessive healthy eating and orthorexic eating tendencies in sport and exercise contexts: a systematic review and meta-analysis. *Journal of Behavioral Addictions, 10*(3), 456–470.

Strahler, J., Wachten, H., Stark, R., & Walter, B. (2021). Alike and different: associations between orthorexic eating behaviors and exercise addiction. *International Journal of Eating Disorders, 54*(8), 1415–1425.

Strahler, J., Wachten, H., Neuhofer, S., & Zimmermann, P. (2022). Psychological correlates of excessive healthy and orthorexic eating: emotion regulation, attachment, and anxious-depressive-stress symptomatology. *Frontiers in Nutrition, 9*, 817047.

Strelau, J., & Zawadzki, B. (2011). Fearfulness and anxiety in research on temperament: temperamental traits are related to anxiety disorders. *Personality and Individual Differences, 50*(7), 907–915.

Stutts L. A. (2020). It's complicated: the relationship between orthorexia and weight/shape concerns, eating behaviors, and mood. *Eating Behaviors, 39*, 101444.

Subhan, F. B., & Chan, C. B. (2016). Review of dietary practices of the 21st century: facts and fallacies. *Canadian Journal of Diabetes, 40*(4), 348–354.

Surís, A., Holliday, R., & North, C. S. (2016). The evolution of the classification of psychiatric disorders. *Behavioral Sciences, 6*(1), 5.

Sutton, S. (2008). *Determinants of Health-Related Behaviours: Theoretical and Methodological Issues.* SAGE Publications Ltd.

Şentürk, E., Güler Şentürk, B., Erus, S., Geniş, B., & Coşar, B. (2022). Dietary patterns and eating behaviors on the border between healthy and pathological orthorexia. *Eating and Weight Disorders, 27*(8), 3279–3288.

Tabri, N., Yung, J. J., & Elliott, C. M. (2022). Connecting a health-focused self-concept with orthorexia nervosa symptoms via fear of losing control over eating unhealthy food and disgust for unhealthy food. *Eating and Weight Disorders, 27*(8), 3569–3578.

Takeda, G.A. (2022). *Ortorexia nervosa, comer intuitivo e comer positivo em nutricionistas, gastrólogos e população geral* [Orthorexia nervosa, intuitive eating and positive eating in dietitians, graduates in gastronomy and general population]. Dissertation, advisor Alvarenga M. dos S. School of Public Health – University of São Paulo. Unpublished thesis.

Talbot, C. V., Campbell, C. E. R., & Greville-Harris, M. (2023). 'Your struggles are valid, you are worthy of help and you deserve to recover': narratives of recovery from orthorexia nervosa. *Eating and Weight Disorders, 28*(1), 25.

Tarsitano, M. G., Pujia, R., Ferro, Y., Mocini, E., Proni, G., Lenzi, F. R., Pujia, A., & Giannetta, E. (2022). Symptoms of orthorexia nervosa are associated with time spent on social media: a web-based survey in an Italian population sample. *European Review for Medical and Pharmacological Sciences, 26*(24), 9327–9335.

Taştekin Ouyaba, A., & Çiçekoğlu Öztürk, P. (2022). The effect of the information-motivation-behavioral skills (IMB) model variables on orthorexia nervosa behaviors of pregnant women. *Eating and Weight Disorders, 27*(1), 361–372.

Telles-Correia, D., Saraiva, S., & Gonçalves, J. (2018). Mental disorder: the need for an accurate definition. *Frontiers in Psychiatry, 9*, 64.

Tena, A., Parra, A., Barajas, M., Bilbao, G. M., Diaz, M. C., Flores, I., et al. (2021). When eating 'correctly' is not so healthy: factor analysis of the ORTO-15 in university students from Mexico City. *Austin Journal of Nutrition & Metabolism, 8*(1), 1100.

Thomas, J. J., Lawson, E. A., Micali, N., Misra, M., Deckersbach, T., & Eddy, K. T. (2017). Avoidant/restrictive food intake disorder: a three-dimensional model of neurobiology with implications for etiology and treatment. *Current Psychiatry Reports, 19*, 1–9.

Thorne, J., Hussain, M., & Mantzios M. (2023). Exploring the relationship between orthorexia nervosa, mindful eating and guilt and shame. *Health Psychology Report, 11*(1), 38–47.

Thorsberg C. (2022). Recognizing orthorexia: the unofficial eating disorder that takes clean and healthy eating too far. https://themessenger.com/grid/recognizing-orthorexia-the-unofficial-eating-disorder-that-takes-clean-and-healthy-eating-too-far.

Thornton, C., & Russell, J. (1997). Obsessive compulsive comorbidity in the dieting disorders. *International Journal of Eating Disorders, 21*(1), 83–87.

Timlin, D., McCormack, J. M., Kerr, M., Keaver, L., & Simpson, E. E. A. (2020). Are dietary interventions with a behaviour change theoretical framework effective in changing dietary patterns? A systematic review. *BMC Public Health, 20*(1), 1857.

Timmerman, G. M., Tahir, M. J., Lewis, R. M., Samoson, D., Temple, H., & Forman, M. R. (2017). Self-management of dietary intake using mindful eating to improve dietary intake for individuals with early stage chronic kidney disease. *Journal of Behavioral Medicine, 40*(5), 702–711.

Toti, E., Cavedon, V., Raguzzini, A., Fedullo, A. L., Milanese, C., Bernardi, E., Bellito, S., Bernardi, M., Sciarra, T., & Peluso, I. (2022). Dietary intakes and food habits of wheelchair basketball athletes compared to gym attendees and individuals who do not practice sport activity. *Endocrine, Metabolic & Immune Disorders Drug Targets, 22*(1), 38–48.

Tremelling, K., Sandon, L., Vega, G. L., & McAdams, C. J. (2017). Orthorexia nervosa and eating disorder symptoms in registered dietitian nutritionists in the United States. *Journal of the Academy of Nutrition and Dietetics*, *117*(10), 1612–1617.

Tucunduva Philippi, S., Guerra, P.H., & Barco Leme, A.C. (2016). Health behavioral theories used to explain dietary behaviors in adolescents: a systematic review. *Nutrire*, *41*, 22.

Turner, P. G., & Lefevre, C. E. (2017). Instagram use is linked to increased symptoms of orthorexia nervosa. *Eating and Weight Disorders*, *22*(2), 277–284.

Uriegas, N. A., Winkelmann, Z. K., Pritchett, K., & Torres-McGehee, T. M. (2021). Examining eating attitudes and behaviors in collegiate athletes, the association between orthorexia nervosa and eating disorders. *Frontiers in Nutrition*, *8*, 763838.

US News and World Report (2023). *Best Diets*. https://health.usnews.com/best-diet/best-diets-overall.

Vaccari, G., Cutino, A., Luisi, F., Giambalvo, N., Navab Daneshmand, S., Pinelli, M., Maina, G., Galeazzi, G. M., Kaleci, S., Albert, U., Atti, A. R., & Ferrari, S. (2021). Is orthorexia nervosa a feature of obsessive–compulsive disorder? A multicentric, controlled study. *Eating and Weight Disorders*, *26*(8), 2531–2544.

Vaillancourt, C., Bédard, A., Bélanger-Gravel, A., Provencher, V., Bégin, C., Desroches, S., & Lemieux, S. (2019). Promoting healthy eating in adults: an evaluation of pleasure-oriented versus health-oriented messages. *Current Developments in Nutrition*, *3*(5), nzz012.

Vainik, U., & Meule, A. (2018). Jangle fallacy epidemic in obesity research: a comment on Ruddock et al. (2017). *International Journal of Obesity*. 2018;42:585–586.

Valente, M., Brenner, R., Cesuroglu, T., Bunders-Aelen, J., & Syurina, E. V. (2020). 'And it snowballed from there': the development of orthorexia nervosa from the perspective of people who self-diagnose. *Appetite*, *155*, 104840.

Valente, M., Renckens, S., Bunders-Aelen, J., & Syurina, E. V. (2022a). The #orthorexia community on Instagram. *Eating and Weight Disorders*, *27*(2), 473–482.

Valente, M., Cesuroglu, T., Labrie, N., & Syurina, E. V. (2022b). 'When Are We Going to Hold Orthorexia to the Same Standard as Anorexia and Bulimia?' Exploring the medicalization process of orthorexia nervosa on Twitter. *Health Communication*, *37*(7), 872–879.

Valente, M., Syurina, E. V., & Donini, L. M. (2019). Shedding light upon various tools to assess orthorexia nervosa: a critical literature review with a systematic search. *Eating and Weight Disorders*, *24*(4), 671–682.

Vandereycken W. (2011). Media hype, diagnostic fad or genuine disorder? Professionals' opinions about night eating syndrome, orthorexia, muscle dysmorphia, and emetophobia. *Eating Disorders*, *19*(2), 145–155.

van Eeden, A. E., van Hoeken, D., & Hoek, H. W. (2021). Incidence, prevalence and mortality of anorexia nervosa and bulimia nervosa. *Current Opinion in Psychiatry*, *34*(6), 515–524.

Vanzhula, I. A., Kinkel-Ram, S. S., & Levinson, C. A. (2021). Perfectionism and difficulty controlling thoughts bridge eating disorder and obsessive-compulsive disorder symptoms: a network analysis. *Journal of Affective Disorders*, *283*, 302–309.

Varga, M., Thege, B. K., Dukay-Szabó, S., Túry, F., & van Furth, E. F. (2014). When eating healthy is not healthy: orthorexia nervosa and its measurement with the ORTO-15 in Hungary. *BMC Psychiatry*, *14*, 59.

Veale D. (2002). Over-valued ideas: a conceptual analysis. *Behaviour Research and Therapy*, *40*(4), 383–400.

Villa, M., Opawsky, N., Manriquez, S., Ananías, N., Vergara-Barra, P., & Leonario-Rodriguez, M. (2022). Orthorexia nervosa risk and associated factors among Chilean nutrition students: a pilot study. *Journal of Eating Disorders*, *10*(1), 6.

Vitousek, K. M., & Brown, K. E. (2015). Cognitive-behavioral theory of eating disorders. In: L. Smolak and M. P. Levine (Eds.). *The Wiley Handbook of Eating Disorders* (pp. 222–237). Wiley-Blackwell.

Vuillier, L., Robertson, S., & Greville-Harris, M. (2020). Orthorexic tendencies are linked with difficulties with emotion identification and regulation. *Journal of Eating Disorders*, *8*, 15.

Wakefield J. C. (2016). Diagnostic issues and controversies in DSM-5: return of the false positives problem. *Annual Review of Clinical Psychology*, *12*, 105–132.

Walker-Swanton, F. E., Hay, P., & Conti, J. E. (2020). Perceived need for treatment associated with orthorexia nervosa symptoms. *Eating Behaviors*, *38*, 101415.

Waller, G., Cordery, H., Corstorphine, E., Hinrichsen, H., Lawson, R., Mountford, V., & Russell, K. (2007). *Cognitive Behavioral Therapy for Eating Disorders: A Comprehensive Treatment Guide*. Cambridge University Press.

Wang, X., & Cheng, Z. (2020). Cross-sectional studies strengths, weaknesses and recommendations. *Chest Journal*, *158*, S65-S71.

Warren, J. M., Smith, N., & Ashwell, M. (2017). A structured literature review on the role of mindfulness, mindful eating and intuitive eating in changing eating behaviours: effectiveness and associated potential mechanisms. *Nutrition Research Reviews, 30*(2), 272–283.

Weinstock, M., & Mazzeo, S. E. (2022). College students' perceptions of individuals following popular diets and individuals with orthorexia nervosa. *Eating Behaviors, 47*, 101671.

White, M., Berry, R., & Rodgers, R. F. (2020). Body image and body change behaviors associated with orthorexia symptoms in males. *Body Image, 34*, 46–50.

White, M., Berry, R., Sharma, A., & Rodgers, R. F. (2021). A qualitative investigation of orthorexia nervosa among US college students: characteristics and sociocultural influences. *Appetite, 162*, 105168.

Wickham, S. R., Amarasekara, N. A., Bartonicek, A., & Conner, T. S. (2020). The big three health behaviors and mental health and well-being among young adults: a cross-sectional investigation of sleep, exercise, and diet. *Frontiers in Psychology, 11*, 579205.

Wild, H., Kyröläinen, A. J., & Kuperman, V. (2022). How representative are student convenience samples? A study of literacy and numeracy skills in 32 countries. *Plos One, 17*(7), e0271191.

Willett, W., Rockström, J., Loken, B., Springmann, M., Lang, T., Vermeulen, S., Garnett, T., Tilman, D., DeClerck, F., Wood, A., Jonell, M., Clark, M., Gordon, L. J., Fanzo, J., Hawkes, C., Zurayk, R., Rivera, J. A., De Vries, W., Majele Sibanda, L., Afshin, A., … & Murray, C. J. L. (2019). Food in the Anthropocene: the EAT-Lancet Commission on healthy diets from sustainable food systems. *Lancet, 393*(10170), 447–492.

Williams, B. M., & Levinson, C. A. (2021). Intolerance of uncertainty and maladaptive perfectionism as maintenance factors for eating disorders and obsessive-compulsive disorder symptoms. *European Eating Disorders Review, 29*(1), 101–111.

Winkens, L., Elstgeest, L., van Strien, T., Penninx, B., Visser, M., & Brouwer, I. A. (2020). Does food intake mediate the association between mindful eating and change in depressive symptoms? *Public Health Nutrition, 23*(9), 1532–1542.

World Health Organization (2018). *Healthy Diet.* Fact Sheet No. 394. www.who.int/mediacentre/factsheets/fs394/en/.

World Health Organization. (2019). *International Statistical Classification of Diseases and Related Health Problems* (11th ed.). https://icd.who.int/.

World Health Organization (2020). *Healthy Diet.* www.who.int/news-room/fact-sheets/detail/healthy-diet.

Yakın, E., Obeid, S., Fekih-Romdhane, F., Soufia, M., Sawma, T., Samaha, S., Mhanna, M., Azzi, R., Mina, A., & Hallit, S. (2022). 'In-between orthorexia' profile: the co-occurrence of pathological and healthy orthorexia among male and female non-clinical adolescents. *Journal of Eating Disorders*, *10*(1), 155.

Yakın, E., Raynal, P., & Chabrol, H. (2022). Distinguishing between healthy and pathological orthorexia: a cluster analytic study. *Eating and Weight Disorders*, 27(1), 325–334.

Yardımcı, H., & Demirer, B. (2022). The effect of orthorexia nervosa on food label reading habits among university students. *Eating and Weight Disorders*, 27(6), 2173–2180.

Yassıbaş, E., & Gençer Bingöl, F. (2023). The relationship between orthorexic tendency and bread consumption habits in adults: a cross-sectional study. *Hacettepe Üniversitesi Sağlık Bilimleri Fakültesi Dergisi*, *10*(2), 365–376.

Yilmaz, F. C. (2023). Orthorexia and eating attitudes in health sciences students. *Nigerian Journal of Clinical Practice*, *26*(4), 502–507.

Yılmaz, M. N., & Dundar, C. (2022). The relationship between orthorexia nervosa, anxiety, and self-esteem: a cross-sectional study in Turkish faculty members. *BMC Psychology*, *10*(1), 82.

Yilmaz, Z., Halvorsen, M., Bryois, J., Yu, D., Thornton, L. M., Zerwas, S., Micali, N., Moessner, R., Burton, C. L., Zai, G., Erdman, L., Kas, M. J., Arnold, P. D., Davis, L. K., Knowles, J. A., Breen, G., Scharf, J. M., Nestadt, G., Mathews, C. A., Bulik, C. M., … Eating Disorders Working Group of the Psychiatric Genomics Consortium, Tourette Syndrome/Obsessive–Compulsive Disorder Working Group of the Psychiatric Genomics Consortium (2020). Examination of the shared genetic basis of anorexia nervosa and obsessive-compulsive disorder. *Molecular Psychiatry*, *25*(9), 2036–2046.

Yılmaz, H., Karakuş, G., Tamam, L., Demirkol, M. E., Namlı, Z., & Yeşiloğlu, C. (2020). Association of orthorexic tendencies with obsessive-compulsive symptoms, eating attitudes and exercise. *Neuropsychiatric Disease and Treatment*, *16*, 3035–3044.

Yoshimura, A., Kusama, Y., Omura, Y., Shibata, M., & Maihara, T. (2023). A case of eating disorder diagnosed as orthorexia nervosa. *Cureus*, *15*(1), e33801.

Yung, J. J., & Tabri, N. (2022). The association of perfectionism, health-focused self-concept, and erroneous beliefs with orthorexia nervosa symptoms: a moderated mediation model. *International Journal of Eating Disorders*, *55*(7), 892–901.

Yurtdaş-Depboylu, G., Kaner, G., & Özçakal, S. (2022). The association between social media addiction and orthorexia nervosa, eating attitudes, and body image among adolescents. *Eating and Weight Disorders*, *27*(8), 3725–3735.

Zakhour, M., Haddad, C., Sacre, H., Tarabay, C., Zeidan, R. K., Akel, M., Hallit, R., Kheir, N., Obeid, S., Salameh, P., & Hallit, S. (2021). Differences in the associations between body dissatisfaction and eating outcomes by gender? A Lebanese population study. *Revue d'Épidémiologie et de Santé Publique, 69*(3), 134–144.

Zagaria, A., Barbaranelli, C., Mocini, E., & Lombardo, C. (2023). Cross-cultural adaptation and psychometric properties of the Italian version of the Orthorexia Nervosa Inventory (ONI). *Journal of Eating Disorders, 11*(1), 144.

Zagaria, A., Vacca, M., Cerolini, S., Ballesio, A., & Lombardo, C. (2022). Associations between orthorexia, disordered eating, and obsessive-compulsive symptoms: a systematic review and meta-analysis. *International Journal of Eating Disorders, 55*(3), 295–312.

Zemlyanskaya, Y., Valente, M., & Syurina, E. V. (2022). Orthorexia nervosa and Instagram: exploring the Russian-speaking conversation around #орторексия. *Eating and Weight disorders, 27*(3), 1011–1020.

Zhou, X., Schneider, S. C., Cepeda, S. L., & Storch, E. A. (2020). Orthorexia nervosa in China: an exploration of phenomenology and clinical corre-lates among university students. *Journal of Cognitive Psychotherapy, 34*(3), 225–241.

Zickgraf H. F. (2020). Re. 'Sex differences in orthorexic eating behaviors: a sys-tematic review and meta-analytical integration'. *Nutrition, 70,* 110571.

Zickgraf, H. F. (2020). Treatment of pathologic healthy eating (orthorexia nervosa). In E. A. Storch, D. McKay, & J. S. Abramowitz (Eds.), *Advanced Casebook of Obsessive-Compulsive and Related Disorders: Conceptualizations and Treatment* (pp. 21–40). Elsevier Academic Press.

Zickgraf, H. F., & Barrada, J. R. (2022). Orthorexia nervosa vs. healthy orth-orexia: relationships with disordered eating, eating behavior, and healthy lifestyle choices. *Eating and Weight Disorders, 27*(4), 1313–1325.

Zickgraf, H. F., & Ellis, J. M. (2018). Initial validation of the Nine Item Avoidant/Restrictive Food Intake disorder screen (NIAS): a measure of three restric-tive eating patterns. *Appetite, 123,* 32–42.

Zickgraf, H. F., Ellis, J. M., & Essayli, J. H. (2019). Disentangling orthorexia ner-vosa from healthy eating and other eating disorder symptoms: relationships with clinical impairment, comorbidity, and self-reported food choices. *Appetite, 134,* 40–49.

Zoghbi, R., Awad, E., Hallit, S., & Matta, C. (2023). Prevalence of orthorexic tendencies and their correlates among Lebanese patients with cancer. *Perceptual and Motor Skills, 130*(5), 1952–1969.

# Index